Equine Sports Coaching

Equine Sports Coaching

Alison Lincoln, BSc Equine Sports Coaching

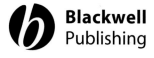

Blackwell
Publishing

This edition first published 2008
© 2008 by Alison Lincoln

Blackwell Publishing was acquired by John Wiley & Sons in February 2007. Blackwell's publishing programme has been merged with Wiley's global Scientific, Technical, and Medical business to form Wiley-Blackwell.

Registered office
John Wiley & Sons Ltd, The Atrium, Southern Gate, Chichester, West Sussex, PO19 8SQ, United Kingdom

Editorial office
9600 Garsington Road, Oxford, OX4 2DQ, United Kingdom

For details of our global editorial offices, for customer services and for information about how to apply for permission to reuse the copyright material in this book please see our website at www.wiley.com/wiley-blackwell.

Library of Congress Cataloging-in-Publication Data
Lincoln, Alison.
  Equine sports coaching / Alison Lincoln.
       p. cm.
   ISBN-13: 978-1-4051-7962-1 (alk. paper)
   ISBN-10: 1-4051-7962-7 (alk. paper)
 1. Horsemanship–Coaching.   I. Title.

SF309.L489 2008
798.2'4071–dc22
                             2007049287

A catalogue record for this book is available from the British Library.

Set in 9.5 on 12 pt Palatino by SNP Best-set Typesetter Ltd., Hong Kong
Printed in Singapore by C.O.S. Printers Pte Ltd

1   2008

Contents

Acknowledgements

Thanks to the University of Worcester for inspiring me to write this book; to Warwickshire College for their continued support; to Wiley-Blackwell for giving me this opportunity; and to David, whose patience and encouragement have been invaluable.

Whilst I have made every possible effort to contact the rights owners of all images used in this book, there have been cases where it has not been possible to trace the relevant parties. If you believe that you are the owner of an image or images used in this book and I have not contacted you prior to publication, please do contact me via the publisher.

Cover photos courtesy of Photo-Synergy.

Introduction

The Coaching Task Force set up by the government in 2002 highlighted the need to develop coaching across all sports. The main concerns identified were that too many unqualified individuals were involved with coaching and there was no national coaching structure. In fact, a study carried out by Sports Coach UK in 2004 identified that approximately 40,000 coaches were active in the U.K. but only 4,990 (1.3%) of them had formal coaching qualifications.

As a result the Task Force recommended the introduction of a UK Coaching Certificate (UKCC), which came into being on 1 January 2007. Thirty-one sports, including equestrian sport and leisure, are involved in this initiative, the objective of which is to advance coach education programmes and support the development of coaching as a career.

In the future any coaching of horses and riders will need to be carried out by qualified individuals. All current BHS registered instructors will need to undergo additional training in order to gain the UKCC qualification, of which there are three levels. Any individual involved in teaching at riding schools, riding club, or Pony Club level, and those involved in the BEF disciplines (British Dressage, British Eventing, British Show Jumping Association, British Equestrian Vaulting, British Reining, British Horse Driving Trials Association, Endurance GB, and Riding for the Disabled) will also need to hold a UKCC endorsed coaching qualification.

This book aims to provide an overview of the many aspects involved in the process of coaching horses and riders and to take techniques that have been researched and used successfully in other sports and make them available to equine coaches. It also hopes to provide a useful reference book for those competitors (amateur or professional) who prefer to coach themselves and are looking to update their knowledge on how they can best prepare themselves and their horses for competition success.

Equine
Sports
Coaching

The Coaching Process

Chapter Objective

To provide an overview of the different approaches to coaching; the purpose, philosophy and role of the coach; and a guide to effective communication and feedback.

1.1 APPROACHES TO COACHING

In the equine industry, there are individuals employed as trainers, instructors, and coaches. But what is the difference between a trainer, an instructor, and a coach, if indeed there is any? Does what you call yourself affect the types of clients you are likely to get? Do potential clients perceive differences between the role of an instructor, a trainer and a coach?

A straw poll of those involved in the industry would probably differentiate the terms as follows.

Instructors:
- tell the rider what to do
- provide lessons that incorporate tried and tested exercises
- focus predominantly on the rider
- are found mainly in riding schools, colleges, and the Pony Club

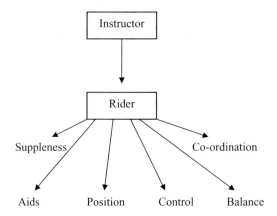

Figure 1.1   Focus of an instructor.

- pass on facts and knowledge
- are viewed as concentrating on improving basic riding skills
- will have instructor qualifications from either the British Horse Society (BHS) or the Association of British Riding Schools (ABRS)
- adopt an authoritarian approach, for example, "Do as I say"

Figure 1.1 illustrates the areas an instructor is likely to focus on in their lessons. They are expected to be experienced and knowledgeable about the steps needed to develop a beginner into a competent rider on the flat and over fences. Instructors are generally associated with the leisure industry, that is, riders who participate for enjoyment and exercise.

Trainers:
- pass on their skills and knowledge by guiding practice
- focus predominantly on the horse
- are viewed as producing horses for competition
- are often freelance
- are perceived as having "hands on" experience
- work in partnership with the rider

Figure 1.2 illustrates the areas a trainer is likely to focus on in their training sessions. Trainers are expected to be able to demonstrate experience and knowledge in producing horses from novice level to established both on the flat and over fences. Trainers are generally associated with the serious amateur, those who may work outside of the horse industry, riding and competing in the evenings and at weekends.

Coaches:
- encourage self-awareness
- work with teams or elite riders in preparation for major competitions
- have often competed at the highest levels themselves
- act as "eyes on the ground"

Figure 1.3 illustrates the areas in which a coach is likely to be interested in when working with horses and riders. Coaches are expected to have a thorough knowledge and experience of developing riders, producing horses, managing teams, and competing. Coaches are generally associated with professional and elite riders, that is, those who make a living from competing or are in contention for national team places.

Interestingly, in other sports (football, hockey, cricket, athletics, swimming, etc.), anybody involved with helping athletes to improve in their chosen sport, whether

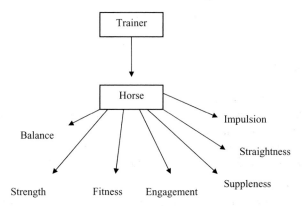

Figure 1.2   Focus of a trainer.

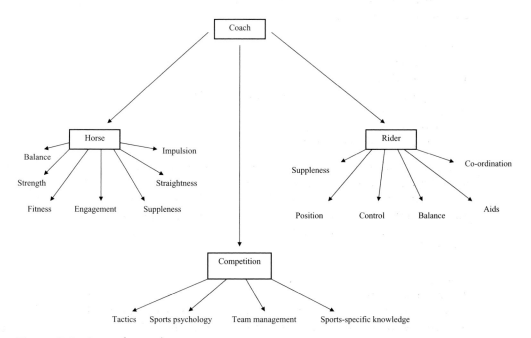

Figure 1.3   Focus of a coach.

for competition or leisure, is referred to as a coach. It is recognised, however, that there are many different approaches to coaching, and these have parallels with the terms commonly used in the equine industry.

Models of Coaching

Lombardo (1999) identified four coaching models:

- Standard (or traditional) model of coaching
- General educational model
- Humanistic model
- Invitational model

Standard Model of Coaching

The standard model of coaching centres on winning. It is a coach-centred approach that does not aspire to educational outcomes such as the growth and development of the individual. It simply aims to improve those areas that will enhance the chance of winning. All decisions are made by the coach, and the individual or team is viewed as belonging to the coach. This approach is more appropriate at the professional or elite level of sport, where team selection, lottery funding, and sponsorship are generally influenced by the success of the rider.

Case Study 1.1

Sally is a former member of the young rider event team and has completed Badminton, Burghley, and Blenheim several times. She now makes her living coaching and runs a training yard in Oxford. Currently, she is coaching an event rider who is aiming to compete at CCI**** (international four-star three-day event) level this year with a view to being selected for the European Championships in two years.

They meet monthly for a two hour coaching session, which comprises dressage and jumping. The sessions focus predominantly on the challenges that the horse and rider will meet in competition and working on issues that the rider has identified in their training or competitions to date. Sally also attends some of the bigger events to help support and assess their performance at competitions.

The riders who will benefit most from this type of coaching are those who require only slight "tweaks" to their technique. They are highly likely to be accomplished producers of horses in their own right. The coach will generally decide which horse is to be selected, what team training must be attended, what the qualifying standard is, and which competitions are compulsory for qualification purposes.

The downside of this approach is that it is not personalised. A rider just breaking into the professional or elite ranks, such as those moving up from Young Riders, are likely to require a higher level of individual support, encouragement, and direction.

General Educational Model

The general educational model, in contrast, focuses on the growth and development of the individual and will typically consist of regular, intense instruction to develop both fitness and skill. The coach remains the primary decision maker. This approach is appropriate in pony clubs, riding schools, and colleges where riders are either being prepared for work within the equine industry or are aiming to improve their general riding skills and where health and safety considerations are paramount.

Case Study 1.2

Tom works at a riding school and has the Assistant Instructor qualification from the BHS. The majority of his clients are children and adults who are learning to ride and attend weekly for a one-hour lesson. The focus of these lessons is for the clients to do as much actual riding as possible in the hour and usually involves Tom setting a number of exercises for them to have a go at. Tom's main objective is that everyone enjoys themselves and stays safe.

The benefit of this model is that the health and well-being of the rider is put first. It is an ideal approach to take with novice riders and children and should emphasise fun, enjoyment, and the acquiring and development of skill. The disadvantage of this approach is that it is unlikely to be as effective for competitive riders who measure their ability and progress against what they have achieved rather than whether they've had a good time.

Humanistic Model of Coaching

The humanistic model is an educational model devoted to the all-round development of the individual. It is rider-centred and focuses on improving the self-awareness of the participant in all areas. Riders are encouraged to reflect on their subjective experiences, and these insights are used to enhance their personal development. The goals of the rider take precedence over those of the coach, whose role is to encourage and support the rider.

The riders are expected to analyse, think, and make important decisions about their learning and aspirations. This approach generally results in the long-term participation of the rider in the sport. The rider-coach relationship is viewed as a co-operative one, although the coach cannot fully relinquish the responsibilities inherent in their position. This is an appropriate approach for coaching in riding clubs and freelance coaching of non-professional competition riders.

Case Study 1.3

Ian is a dressage rider who uses his freelance coaching to support his competing. He has a number of clients who are enthusiastic, non-professional dressage riders. Typically, they attend a one-hour session every couple of weeks. The focus for these sessions is on the progressive development of the horse. The riders are encouraged to reflect on their competition results and identify areas they would like to work on in each session. Ian spends time at the start discussing the focus for the next hour and agrees upon a plan of action with the rider. The exercises are attempted, and Ian provides feedback to help improve the rider's awareness of the effect of the exercise.

The advantage of this approach is that the rider is required to be fully involved and engaged in the whole process. The coach helps them take responsibility for their own development and provides them with the skills to coach themselves when they are not with the coach. This approach is appropriate for most situations, although it may need to be adapted for younger children who have not yet fully developed the ability to analyse and evaluate themselves.

Invitational Model of Coaching

The invitational model focuses on the positive encouragement of all participants. It is characterised by sincere optimism for the riders, trust in their ability, and respect for all individuals connected with the sporting experience, such as parents or other family members. This approach aims to ensure all aspects of the riding experience are inviting, including the people running the coaching sessions, the policies, processes and procedures, the environment, and the facilities. It is designed to increase participation in the sport and is rider-centred, being predominantly concerned with learning and development rather than winning. This approach is appropriate for all organisations involved in the leisure riding industry such as riding schools, riding clubs, pony clubs, and equestrian centres.

Case Study 1.4

Elaine runs an equestrian centre that has close links with the local riding club. She runs weekly dressage and jumping sessions that are open to everyone. The centre has a small café, and those attending the sessions often arrive early to share a cup of coffee and chat with Elaine. The focus of the session is on enjoyment and the positive encouragement of all who attend, most of whom are adults riding for pleasure. The majority do compete in the shows held at the centre and local riding club competitions. Each person knows the others by name, and friends and family members are encouraged to attend as spectators. The atmosphere is relaxed and informal.

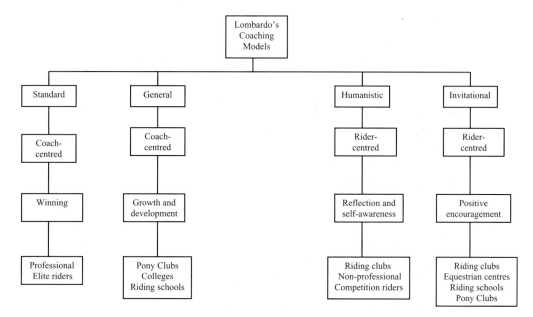

Figure 1.4   Models of coaching.

In reality neither one of these approaches is better or more successful than another, and the experienced coach will be able to recognise which is the most appropriate to adopt given the situation and the individuals they are coaching. Figure 1.4 provides a summary of the four coaching models.

Regardless of their approach, a coach will inevitably find themselves fulfilling a wide range of roles throughout their career (Table 1.1). Whatever role, the purpose of coaching remains the same – the development of the physical and psychological skills required to ride, as well as the wider personal development of the rider. In order to achieve this and remain true to their own values, beliefs, and goals, the coach will need a clearly defined personal coaching philosophy.

1.2   COACHING PHILOSOPHY

The reasons for entering into a career coaching riders are numerous:

- Making a living
- Supporting one's own competing
- Loving the sport
- Wanting to teach
- Working with children
- Traveling
- Gaining reputation and recognition
- Working with horses

Table 1.1. Some of the roles required of a coach.

Instructor	Being able to tell riders how to perform particular skills (e.g., a transition from trot to canter).
Trainer	Being knowledgeable in all aspects that may influence riding success (e.g., nutrition, fitness, training programmes, and competition rules).
Organiser	Ability to organise sessions that meet the needs of those attending (e.g., facilities, equipment, appropriate horses, exercises/activities).
Role model	Act as a role model to children, novices, and those new to riding (e.g., in manner, horsemanship, language, dress, and behaviour).
Judge	Provide simulated competition sessions and therefore be familiar with the rules of each discipline and have an understanding of judging in dressage, show jumping, and fence judging in cross country.
Psychologist	Being able to influence the rider's mental attitude to riding and competing and boost their confidence and motivation in their coaching sessions.
Advisor	Be able to advise riders on their training and competition programmes, care of their horse, and suitable tack and equipment.
Counsellor	Be able to recognise and help resolve problems that may or may not be directly related to riding.
Disciplinarian	Encourage good discipline and implement appropriate consequences of poor discipline.
Referrer	Be able to recognise when additional expertise should be sought and be able to recommend who and where this help can be obtained.
Chauffeur	Transporting horses and riders to events.
Demonstrator	Being able to provide demonstrations to illustrate key skills or concepts.
Mentor	When riders attend sessions, the coach is responsible for their safety and security. Their health and safety should be monitored whilst training and support provided if they have problems or injuries.
Supporter	Provide support at competitions, selection days, or the purchase of a new horse.
Educator	Educate those being coached on ethical behaviour, sportsmanship, and the physical and psychological welfare of the horse.

- Helping riders to develop
- Helping riders get the best from their horses
- Achieving competition success

Research has shown that the common reasons cited by coaches for getting involved with coaching in their chosen sport range from being a natural progression after a competitive career, to being an interested parent or relative, wanting to help young people and others, and to contribute to the sport (Lyle et al, 1997).

Whatever the coach's reasons, it is important to acknowledge them and identify the main priorities and objectives for their coaching practice as this will allow the best career decisions to be made. It is appropriate for a coach to seek their own fulfilment as long as it is not achieved at the rider's or horse's expense. Indeed, the most effective coaches have objectives for themselves, their rider's development, the horse's development, and separate objectives for any competitions being entered.

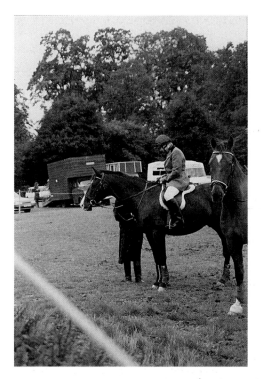

Figure 1.5   It is always nice to win, but a rider's success should not depend on the outcome of an event.

Whatever type or level of rider the coach is working with and whatever their own personal aims and objectives, the overriding principles when coaching should be:

- Winning isn't everything. It can be an important goal, but it is not the most important goal. The welfare of the horse and rider is paramount.
- Losing is not the same thing as failing. Riders should not view losing as a sign of failure.
- Success is not equivalent to winning. Success or failure should not be dependent on the outcome of an event (Figure 1.5).
- Riders should be taught that they are never losers if they give maximum effort. (Smoll and Smith, 2001)

This can be challenging in an environment where reputation, lottery funding, team selection, and sponsorship are heavily based on successful performance.

Qualities of a Coach

Coaches should aim to develop individuals who can think for themselves, analyse situations, and respond appropriately, independently, and wisely. Many studies have been conducted in an attempt to identify the qualities required to be able to do this.

Housner and Griffey (1985) found that experienced coaches were generally more concerned with the skill development of those they coach than novice coaches, who tended to focus more on ensuring their students were active, content, and obedient.

Hardin (1999) and Valle and Bloom (2005) identified that expert, successful coaches across a wide range of sports all had a number of things in common: the ability to select the most appropriate leadership behaviours according to the situation; a personal desire to foster the individual's growth; thorough organisational skills to plan and prepare sessions; and a strong sense of their own goals, philosophy, and personality.

When asked, athletes in a wide variety of sports indicated that they preferred a coach who:

- is fair
- has no favourites
- keeps good control
- gives no extreme punishments
- explains and helps
- gives interesting lessons
- is cheerful, friendly, patient, and understanding
- has a good sense of humour
- takes an interest in the students as individuals

Interestingly, in all this research, winning was not mentioned. This suggests that although winning is important, providing athletes (riders included) feel they are improving and enjoying themselves in a supportive and challenging environment, they will remain satisfied.

The public perception is that good coaching is crucial for top sports people to be successful, it improves people's enjoyment of their sport and increases participation levels (Sports Coach UK, 2004).

Responsibilities of a Coach

Inherent in any coaching is a position of responsibility, not only to the health and safety of every horse and rider but also to the effect a coach can have on riders by what they say and do.

A coach's expectations can have a profound impact on the progress of a rider (Figure 1.6). Children (particularly those under the age of 10) and riders who are very dependent on the coach's feedback are most likely to be influenced by their coach's expectations of them. Strong predictors of a coach's tendency to affect riders

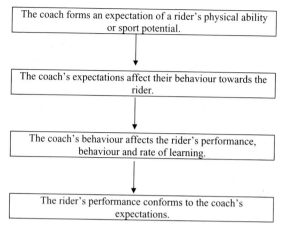

Figure 1.6 Implications of a coach's expectations.

through their own expectations are the level of a coach's own self-reflection and perceived control over their rider's performances (Sternberg Horn et al, 2001).

The coach who believes what they say and do has a direct impact on those they coach are often much better at reflecting on the effect they have on the riders. Those who believe they only provide information and guidance, with it being up to the riders themselves to act on it, are unlikely to reflect on, or take responsibility for, the impact they have and are therefore those most at risk of adversely affecting the riders they coach.

Case Study 1.5

Jenny is running a cross country session for a local pony club. The District Commissioner has advised her that two of the riders (Christopher and Jane) were on the eventing team last year and that Christopher is particularly talented. She implies that Jane was only on the team because her mother was the team selector. During the warm-up session, Jane comes in too fast to a fence and her pony stops. Jenny has developed the expectation that Jane is not a talented rider and sees this stop as proof of her lack of ability. Jenny, therefore, responds by telling Jane to slow down and prepare better. The next rider to attempt the fence is Christopher. His horse also stops, but because Jenny believes him to be a talented rider, she assumes that the pony is just being naughty and tells him to give him a kick and try again.

Later in the session, the group are at the coffin fence, taking it in turns to jump through. When it is his turn, Christopher negotiates the coffin successfully and Jenny responds with approval but stops the others from continuing so she can give Christopher further pointers about approaching the fence. When it is Jane's turn, she also negotiates the fence successfully, and Jenny responds with approval only ("well-ridden, Jane") and lets the group continue taking turns at the fence.

At the water jump towards the end of the course, both Jane and Christopher jump through boldly, but the next two riders have problems. Jenny asks Christopher to provide a lead for these horses at their next three attempts while Jane stands and watches.

In this case study, it is obvious to the outside observer that Jane is receiving less-effective coaching. As a result she is unlikely to show the same skill development as some of the others. In addition, the quality of coaching a rider receives can influence their perception of how competent or skilful the coach thinks they are. If they perceive the coach's view is that they are not as competent or skilful, it can lead to them having lower expectations themselves and an increased level of anxiety.

It is a coach's responsibility to remain aware of the effect of their behaviour towards those they are coaching. Attributing a rider's success to their actions is likely to lead to a rider who develops a high expectancy for future success and a positive attitude towards the sport and their ability to influence the horse. Attributing successful performance to luck ("you were lucky that pole stayed up") or to the horse ("what a good horse for helping you out there") results in a rider who lacks the belief that they can attain the same performance in the future.

Sternberg Horn et al (2001) offered the following recommendations for coaches to help evaluate and modify their behaviour in coaching situations:

- Determine which sources of information you will use to form expectations for each rider (such as those needed to group riders into ability level).
- Realise that the initial assessment may be inaccurate and remain flexible enough to recognise this and take appropriate action.
- Keep a mental tally of how much practice each individual is getting during group coaching sessions.
- Design sessions that provide all riders with the opportunity to improve their skills. This may mean setting different objectives for each rider based on the horse they are riding or the goal they are aiming for.
- Respond to errors with corrective instructions that tell the rider what they can do to improve.
- Evaluate and praise riders on their improvement in skill rather than absolute performance (e.g., "good, straight approach" rather than "well ridden"). This allows the coach to convey the attitude that all riders can improve their skills no matter what level they are currently riding.

1.3 COACHING STYLES

The question is often asked, which style of coaching is the most effective for consistently producing optimal performance? It is actually impossible to give a definitive answer to this because of the wide variety of riders' needs, depending on their

Table 1.2. Coaching styles.

Coach-Centred Approach	Rider-Centred Approach
The coach makes the decisions and directs the ridden exercises.	The emphasis is on the interaction between coach and rider when making decisions.

Table 1.3. Coach-centred approaches.

Autocratic 1	Autocratic 2
• The coach decides on what is done in each session. • Riders are not involved in the decision making. • The coach tells the riders what to do and how to do it. • The coach demands perfect behaviour at all times. • There is a high level of control from the coach. • The coach has a tendency to shout at mistakes/errors/bad behaviour.	• The coach decides on what is done in each session. • Riders are not involved in the decision making. • The coach explains the objective of the session and what is required from the rider in order to achieve this objective. • The riders are encouraged to ask questions. • The coach tells the rider what to do and how to do it.
Consultative 1	**Consultative 2**
• The coach consults with riders about what they think should be done in the session. • The coach decides on what is to be done, which may or may not reflect the thoughts and opinions of the rider.	• The coach consults with a number of people, for example, rider, parent, team selector, etc. • The coach decides what is to be done, which may or may not reflect the thoughts and opinions of those consulted.

discipline, competition level, and experience, and this is before the needs of the horse are considered. It is possible to provide the coach with information on the various options available to them so they can select the most appropriate style for the situation and the horse and rider combination they are coaching.

Coaching styles can be roughly generalised into two distinct approaches – the coach-centred approach and the rider-centred approach (Table 1.2).

These categories can be further subdivided into four coach-centred approaches (autocratic 1 and 2 and consultative 1 and 2) and two rider-centred approaches (participative 1 and 2) to illustrate the different characteristics demonstrated by each style of coach, as shown in Table 1.3 (Chelladurai and Trail, 2001).

Coach-Centred Approach

The coach-centred approach has also been called a task-centred approach because the focus of the coaching is on what has to be done; that is, the needs of the individual are less important then the achievement of goals.

These types of approaches are particularly good when the health and safety of the horse and rider are of paramount concern, such as when coaching in a pony club, college, or riding school environment. On the down side, it is a physically tiring coaching style, and at its worst can intimidate the quieter or less confident rider.

Case Study 1.6

Andy is a coach who works at a local college as well as doing some freelance coaching.

His first coaching session of the day is with a group of Higher National Diploma (HND) students at the college who are working towards their BHS stage 3 riding exam. Andy has already allocated the horses to the students based on their experience, confidence, and ability. He explains that the objective of the session is to ride 5-metre loops in walk, trot, and canter. First, they will practice riding 3-metre loops in each pace and then progress to the 5-metre loops. He gives clear instructions on how to ride the loops and then asks the students if they have any questions before beginning in walk. *Autocratic 2.*

At lunchtime Andy has an individual coaching session with a talented student who has qualified for the Novice Regional Dressage Finals. This student was referred to Andy by another lecturer at the college, who explained that they were having problems with the lengthening and the reasons they felt this was happening. While the student is tacking up in preparation for the session, Andy has a chat with her and her mother about their aspirations, any issues or problems they are encountering, and what they feel would be useful to work on in the session. After watching the rider warm up, Andy suggests they spend some time on a couple of exercises to get the horse working more in front of the leg, which should help improve the overall test marks as well as improving the lengthening. *Consultative 2.*

The final session of the day is an evening show jumping session with a group from the local riding club. Andy spends the first 10 minutes as they warm up talking to the riders individually to find out their experience, any issues or problems, and any particular areas they would like to work on. At the end of the 10 minutes, Andy calls all the riders into the centre of the arena and suggests that they start by working over trotting poles and then progress to grid work to work on the riders' position. *Consultative 1.*

Coaches who adopt the task-centred approach to coaching often exhibit the following characteristics:

- A tendency to develop expectations of a rider.
- A need to demonstrate their own personal authority by making all the decisions. and having strict rules.
- A tendency to demand strict compliance to the rules that are set.
- A tendency to remain emotionally distant from their riders.
- A desire to avoid unstructured situations.

Table 1.4. Rider-centred approaches.

Participative 1	Participative 2
• The coach identifies the objective of the session.	• The coach identifies the objective of the session.
• The rider suggests suitable exercises to achieve the objective.	• The rider suggests exercises and then decides on which will best meet the objective.
• The coach selects the most appropriate exercises.	• The coach sets the health and safety ground rules.
• The coach decides what to do and how to do it.	• The rider decides what to do.
	• The coach gives advice on how to do it.

- A higher need for social approval.
- A tendency to adopt the "this is how I was coached" attitude (Chelladurai and Saleh, 1980).

Rider-Centred Approach

The main rider-centred approach is the participative style in which the coach and the rider make decisions collectively (Table 1.4).

Coaches who adopt the rider-centred approach to coaching often demonstrate the following characteristics:

- An interest in the opinions of the rider and anyone involved with the rider (e.g., parent, partner, sponsor, owner, etc.).
- A respect for the views of the rider and anyone involved with the rider.
- A low likelihood of acting in expectancy-based ways.
- A desire to involve the rider as much as possible in decision making.
- A strong emphasis on good interpersonal relationships with the rider and anyone involved with the rider.
- A willingness to sacrifice success for the good of the rider or horse
(Chelladurai and Saleh, 1980).

Case Study 1.7

Jill is an event rider and qualified coach who is employed by a college on a part-time basis to coach the eventing team. Her remit is to prepare the students for an upcoming competition. In this session they are going to use the show jumps in the arena to practice riding different types of cross country fences. She starts the session by informing the students of the objective and then asking them to suggest how the show jumps could be used to simulate cross country fences. The students make a number of suggestions, and she selects the most appropriate ones and builds the course accordingly. *Participative 1.*

Jill is also involved in training riders to get their coaching qualifications. In this session the riders are looking at how to ride a course of show jumps. Jill has set up a number of fences in the arena. After they warm up and jump a few practice fences, Jill asks the riders to line up in the centre of the arena and suggest how these fences could be best jumped as a course. Each rider must decide on the course they are going to jump and must include all the fences. Jill discusses the route they are going to take with each individual rider to ensure it is safe and sensible. She then asks each rider to jump their course. Once each rider has had a go, all riders return to the centre of the arena to discuss the advantages and disadvantages of each route. *Participative 2.*

As illustrated by the case studies, good coaches are able to adapt their style to fit the needs of the riders they are coaching. This may mean being tough and demanding on some and more encouraging to others. The more the coach can match their own behaviour with the expectations and preferences of the rider and the specific demands of the situation, the greater the rider's satisfaction, enjoyment, and performance.

Interestingly, research has shown that individuals (as opposed to teams) prefer a more person-orientated approach, males tolerate an authoritarian coach more than females, and winning apparently makes little difference to children, although they know it is important to adults. In reality, the experience, maturity, and skill level of each rider is likely to influence the selection of the most appropriate coaching style (Smith and Smoll, 1997).

In fact, although this section has discussed coaching styles, they could equally be termed decision-making styles because all activities carried out by a coach involve some form of decision making; decisions such as which exercises will best help the horse and rider to progress or which horse is best suited to which rider in a riding school setting are made continually.

Using this terminology provides the coach with a useful insight into the purpose of coaching, especially when it is considered that decision making can be defined as the process of selecting one alternative from many choices in order to achieve a desired outcome. The implication is that effective decision making and therefore effective coaching is determined by the nature of the problem or situation rather than the personality of the coach (Chelladurai and Trail, 2001).

Being able to assess the best approach for the situation is a key skill required for effective coaching. However, once the most appropriate approach has been identified, other skills will be needed in order to implement it successfully.

The autocratic style requires someone who is able to identify alternatives, evaluate each alternative individually, and then select the best option for achieving the desired outcome. The participative style requires someone who is able to act as a facilitator and discussion leader. They must be able to articulate the problem or issue clearly and assist those involved in reaching a good decision. This often means remaining as impartial as possible.

So, in answer to the question regarding which style of coaching is the most effective for consistently producing optimal performance, perhaps the best way to judge a coach's effectiveness is to look at the riders themselves and ask the following questions:

- Are they reaching their potential?
- Are they learning and progressing?
- Are they achieving their goals?

(Murray and Mann, 2001)

1.4 COMMUNICATION AND FEEDBACK

Fundamentally, coaching relies on effective communication between coach and rider. The rider must not only receive the information being given but also understand it. This means using appropriate vocabulary for the age and experience of the riders and avoiding jargon or overly technical instructions.

How these instructions or explanations are given is also important. They should be brief and to the point, with the coach speaking slower than in normal conversation and including pauses to provide the opportunity for the information to be absorbed.

Random questions can be used to check for understanding. Rather than simply asking "is that clear?" or "does everybody understand?", use open questions such as "so, when you get to A what do you need to do?" or "talk me through the aids you are going to use". If necessary be prepared to repeat or reword the instructions.

Simple guidelines are:
- Give the instructions clearly and concisely.
- Check for understanding, using open questions.
- Let the rider(s) get on with it.

Terminology

Closed questions elicit one word answers such as "yes" or "no".
Example: Did you enjoy the coaching session today?

Open questions provide scope for more detailed answers.
Example: What did you enjoy about the coaching session today?

Group coaching presents its own challenges in terms of verbal communication. The aim should be to face the riders at all times and direct the voice at everyone. This may mean that the coach needs to adjust their position frequently.

The voice is a powerful tool and can be used to stimulate the group by varying the volume, tone, pitch, pace, and emphasis. Consider the following example.

Different words in the sentence are emphasised to demonstrate how emphasis will alter the meaning (it works best if read aloud).

1. "I **can't** believe this is happening to me."
2. "I can't **believe** this is happening to me."
3. "I can't believe **this** is happening to me."
4. "I can't believe this is happening to **me.**"

Sentence one and three sound quite negative, as if something bad or unwanted is happening to the person. Sentences two and four have a slightly incredulous quality to them, with the emphasis on **believe** and **me** suggesting that it might be something good and unexpected that has happened. The coach can use these changes of emphasis to highlight key words or key actions that the riders should focus on.

The coach can use the volume of their voice to get attention, but not simply through raising their voice or shouting. Often the most effective means of ensuring that riders stop talking is to drop the volume. In general, people are innately curious, and the sound of a lowered voice (especially if their expectation is to get shouted at) can pique their curiosity about what is being said, thus talking will stop in order to hear what is being discussed.

The tone in which instructions or information is given is very important, particularly with riders who are not familiar with the coach and their style. This is because it is the tone of what is said rather than the words that are said that can convey disapproval, disappointment, enthusiasm, and encouragement. Sarcasm should be avoided.

The pitch and pace of a coach's voice can be used to influence the energy levels of the rider. Reducing the speed and lowering the pitch of what is being said can help to calm and relax overexcited riders, whereas increasing the speed and pitch can help to energise laid-back riders.

Not all communication is verbal. Non-verbal communication can be as powerful and potentially as confusing. Consider the coach who is talking to Pony Club members at their summer camp on the importance of being fit to ride. What the coach is saying sounds both reasonable and important; however, the coach is clearly overweight and therefore their words appear contrary to their actions. This kind of confusion diminishes the effect of the information being given. In essence coaches should "walk the talk" – or at least the message they are conveying non-verbally should match the message they are conveying verbally.

Other forms of non-verbal communication can lend weight to what is being said or communicate information or feedback when the voice can't be heard. Arm movements such as clapping can provide visual evidence of approval; facial expressions can be used to convey confusion, disappointment, or delight; posture can indicate enthusiasm or boredom; and eye contact helps to make the information being conveyed personal to the individual – as well as letting any distracted pony clubbers know the coach has an eye on them! Table 1.5 gives examples of using both verbal and non-verbal communication.

Table 1.5. Using verbal and non-verbal communication.

Non-Verbal Communication	Verbal Communication
Establish and maintain eye contact.	Paraphrase and summarise what is said to clarify and check understanding.
Use gestures (such as head nodding) to indicate that attention is being paid to what is being said.	Use verbal encouragement to keep the person talking such as "uh-huh" or "I understand"
Avoid defensive gestures, such as crossing arms and legs or leaning away from the person talking.	Use open questions – avoid using "why", as this can be seen as defensive.
Give enough "wait" time for questions to be processed or considered.	Use reflection – "it must be exciting when . . .", "It must have been hard to . . ."

Table 1.6. Listening styles.

Active Listening	The listener is concerned about the content, intent, and feelings of the message being transmitted and is genuinely interested in the person talking.
Superficial/Inattentive	The listener tunes out quickly once they think there is enough information to decipher the speaker's intent. Often they fail to comprehend the underlying message.
Arrogant	The listener is more interested in what they have to say in reply rather than what the other person is saying. The listener waits for the pause so they can jump in.

Listening

The other aspect to effective communication is listening. This is not only the ability to hear and interpret what is being said, but also to decipher the underlying meaning (or what is not being said) of the person talking. Smith (2001) identified three types of listening: active listening, superficial/inattentive listening, and arrogant listening (Table 1.6).

Arrogant listening is characterised by the person looking for the pause in the other person's talking in order to jump in with their own thought and opinions. Superficial or inattentive listening is characterised by the person listening to the first part of what is being said and then assuming they know what is coming next so they tune out. Active listening is characterised by the person taking an active interest in what is being said by asking questions and clarifying the thoughts and ideas. Effective communication relies on developing active listening skills and the ability to understand and communicate messages both verbally and non-verbally.

Potential Barriers to Communication

Information overload is a common mistake made by many coaches. Often the initial instruction is followed up by a few do's and don'ts as well as possible contingencies if something goes wrong. Once the rider has set out to ride the exercise, even more instructions or corrections are issued.

The coach should aim to give precise instructions, let the riders attempt the exercise, and refrain from issuing further instructions until the rider has completed the task. This not only prevents over-reliance of the rider on the coach but also helps to increase their own self-awareness, especially if there is the expectation of a discussion after the exercise.

Ordering, directing, or telling a rider what to do inhibits two-way communication. The rider is likely to be reluctant to ask any questions. They will rely heavily on the coach to resolve any problems or issues, they won't develop the self-awareness necessary to make corrections, and they are likely to lose confidence in their own ability to improve without the input of the coach.

Other possible barriers include:
- The rider may jump to a conclusion before having fully heard and understood the instructions, particularly if the exercise is a familiar one.
- The rider may lack the motivation to listen or convert the instructions into action.
- The coach may have difficulty expressing what they want to say.
- Emotions may interfere in the communication process.
- There may be a clash of personality.
- The coach may be prone to preaching or moralising.

(Smith, 2001)

Feedback

The coach's job is to provide an environment that is encouraging and supportive. To do this, a coach should give positive feedback first (catch them doing something right), then suggest ways of improving. A coach should never openly use negative feedback such as "you didn't do...", "good but...", "that was wrong because...".

Pieron and Goncalves (1987) identified that experienced coaches used positive prescriptive feedback more frequently than less experienced or less successful coaches whose use of negative prescriptive feedback was more prevalent.

Terminology

Positive prescriptive feedback entails praising what has been done well and suggesting specific improvements and things to do next.
Example: Well ridden on the turn. Next time try waiting for the fence to come to you.

Negative prescriptive feedback occurs when a rider is criticised and told not to do something.
Example: You turned in too tight, and next time don't chase into the fence.

Feedback has been shown to have the single biggest impact on the quality of learning, more than any other factor. This is because for learning to take place, the rider needs to know what they are aiming at, the level at which they are currently performing, and how to close the gap between the two. The traditional method of providing feedback is the coach telling the rider what they have done right or wrong and what they need to do differently. However, the emerging consensus is that this may not be the most effective way to provide feedback as it relies heavily on the input of the coach and does not involve the rider sufficiently.

Feedback Strategies

There are many different ways for riders to receive feedback. Some are directly instigated by the coach, and some are simply facilitated by the coach, such as peer assessment, peer explaining, and self-assessment.

Terminology

Peer assessment is when riders of the same level, age, or experience give feedback to each other.

Peer explaining is when the riders in the group are asked to explain how to do something or explain the exercise the coach has just set.

Self-assessment is when the rider is asked to comment on or evaluate their own performance.

Peer assessment can be used when coaching a group of adults or older children. It encourages all members of the group to engage in the exercise and actively watch when others are performing.

Case Study 1.8

Nick is running a show jumping rally for the local Pony Club. After some initial warming up on the flat and over a grid, the group is called into the middle of the arena while Nick sets up a course of jumps. He explains that each rider will jump the course, and then the others in the group will provide feedback on how they have done.

Specifically, he asks the group to assess each individual on how straight the approach was to each fence and whether the horse was being ridden forwards enough into the fences. He asks the group to give each rider an overall mark out of 10 and that this should not be based on whether the horse knocks a pole down or stops but whether the rider has ridden straight and forward to the fences. The person who had just jumped the course was also asked to rate themselves against the same criteria.

The first rider to jump the course is Ann. After she has completed it, Nick asks her for her own assessment, and she awards herself 5 out of 10 as she felt her turn into fence 4 was too tight and she had a fence down in the double. The others in the group award her 7 or 8 out of 10 and comment that although the fence came down, she had ridden straight and forward into the double and was unlucky to drop the pole. Nick then summarises the feedback and the scores and suggests how Ann could improve her round next time.

After the rally, Nick comments to one of the parents how useful he finds this type of feedback. He says that invariably the other members of the group are very positive when giving feedback, and it helps him to get them to focus on the process of riding a course of show jumps rather than the outcome, that is, whether they had incurred faults. He reflects that they all appear to come away feeling more successful and in control of their own performances because of this approach.

Peer explaining is a variation on peer assessment and is a less risky approach because it is impersonal. Initially, it can be as basic as asking for a volunteer to explain the aids for canter. For more advanced riders it could be explaining what is meant by impulsion or how to increase engagement in downward transitions. One of the benefits of peer explaining is that it can also act as an aid for the coach to assess the riders' understanding of an exercise or highlight areas which need more attention.

Case Study 1.9

Ben is taking a riding club flatwork session for those aiming to compete at Pre-liminary level. The group has warmed up in walk and trot and then been called in to the centre of the arena to allow everybody to canter individually. Ben explains that the exercise is to establish trot around the arena, and when they are ready, to go onto a 20-metre circle at A or C and ask for canter. Then they will canter down the long side before going onto another 20-metre circle at the other end and doing a transition to trot.

Before sending out the first person, he asks the group, "what are the aids to canter?", followed by, "what do you think is important to be able to carry out this exercise?" He then summarises the answers he gets and adds anything that has been missed.

He asks for a volunteer to go first. Sheila says she'll have a go. Before she starts, Ben asks her to talk him through how she is going to ride the exercise, including the aids for canter. She then attempts the exercise and returns to the group.

Each rider in the group goes through the same process. When it is their turn, they are asked by Ben the same question related to their horse: "Talk me through how you are going to ride this exercise, including the aids for canter." This makes it personal to the individual, helps to clarify in the rider's mind what they are going to do, how they are going to do it, and when. It also helps Ben to ensure that everybody understands what needs to be done and how to do it.

It is a particularly useful method for checking that everybody knows the aids (in this instance to canter) without actually asking them outright, which might be embarrassing if the rider gets it wrong or has to admit they don't know. It also means that if a rider has not absorbed the instructions fully, they have the opportunity to hear others explain it and then clarify it in their own words.

Self-assessment is simply asking the rider to analyse their own performance and make suggestions about how to improve it. The benefit of this approach is that it encourages the rider to take responsibility for their own learning by increasing their self-awareness and their ability to evaluate where they need to make changes. It also helps to create the belief that improvement is possible and within the rider's control.

Case Study 1.10

Leah is coaching Lucy, who has had some problems on cross country courses with offset combinations. For this session Leah has set up a course of show jumps around the jumping paddock, which includes several offset combinations. After warming up on the flat and over a couple of practice fences, Leah asks Lucy to jump the course and then come back to discuss it.

After completing the course, Leah asks Lucy the following questions to encourage her to evaluate her own performance and identify where improvements could be made:

- How did that go?
  It was OK I guess.
- What went well?
  Well, we had quite good rhythm and got good turns into 5 and 6.
- What were you pleased with?
  I was actually pleased that we got through the offset combination without knocking it down.

- What didn't go so well?
  I still felt we just scrambled through it. If it was bigger we may have been in trouble.
- Anything you would do differently?
  I probably need to shorten the canter more before the combination and ride straight through the jumps rather than trying to fiddle about between them to get straight.
- How confident do you feel about jumping offset combinations?
  Not hugely.
- What would make you feel more confident?
  Well, I noticed that quite a few people in the warm up ring were jumping the practice fences at angles off both reins, and I thought that might be worth doing so we get used to jumping on the angle.
- What do you think is important when jumping offset combinations?
  Probably to get a direct line through the two fences and then go for it.

This is a very useful approach for the more experienced rider as it facilitates them finding the solution or at least identifying potential strategies to help solve the problem. If Leah felt that Lucy was missing something, she could use questions such as, "have you considered . . . ?", "do you think . . . might help?", "what would happen if you tried . . . ?", or "it looks to me as if . . . What do you think?"

Clearly, these approaches rely on the coach's ability to ask thought provoking, open questions that require more than a one- or two-word answer and that challenge riders to think about and express their opinions. Equally, these types of questions can be effectively used to check understanding and diagnose areas that may require further explanation.

The traditional approach of providing direct feedback to riders should not, however, be discarded. It has an important role to play in developing self-esteem and self-image. A well-timed "well-ridden" or "good riding" can make a rider's day (Figure 1.7). The coach has both the privilege and the responsibility to help riders develop their views of themselves, and this can have a huge impact on their development in other areas of their life. Thus, it is important to ensure that as a coach you have a positive impact by:

- Knowing the first names of all the riders being coached.
- Identifying several different ways of conveying praise, both verbal (well done, that's right, good riding) and non-verbal (clapping, nodding the head, smiling).
- Praising effort first, as this is in the rider's complete control, and results second.
- Approaching coaching with energy and enthusiasm.

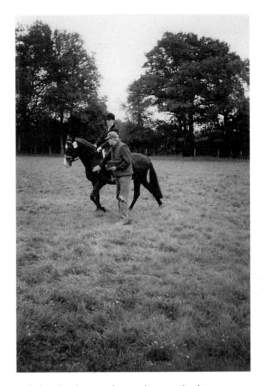

Figure 1.7 Well-timed feedback can have the single biggest impact on learning and performance.

Feedback and Reinforcement

Feedback can serve as reinforcement (positive or negative) or punishment for a particular action or behaviour. Reinforcement aims to increase the likelihood of a rider repeating a behaviour or action by either praising the behaviour (positive reinforcement) when it occurs or by making the consequences (negative reinforcement) of not performing the behaviour unpleasant or undesirable. Punishment aims to decrease the likelihood of the behaviour being repeated by punishing it when it occurs.

Case Study 1.11

The equine students at a college know that if they turn up late for their morning stable duties the yard manager will take away their riding privileges on the weekend. To avoid this happening (as they all like to hack out over the weekend) they ensure their alarm clocks are set and turn up 5 minutes early. *Negative reinforcement*.

A college student is repeatedly late for a show jumping session after lunch. When they do turn up, the coach criticises them in front of the whole group for being late and informs them that as a result they will have to put all the show jumps away on their own at the end of the session. *Punishment*.

At the end of the day a college student returns to the yard, even though they are not scheduled for duties, to brush off the sweat marks from the horses that were used in the afternoon sessions. She had noticed the previous day that although washed off, they had not been brushed to remove marks before being put to bed. The yard manager notices this, thanks the student, and comments to her year tutor about her commitment to the horses well-being. The year tutor subsequently also praises the rider in her next tutorial. *Positive reinforcement*.

The positive approach is designed to strengthen the desired behaviours by motivating riders to perform them again. The negative approach attempts to eliminate unwanted behaviour by motivating riders to avoid the consequences of the behaviour or action. Unfortunately, this approach is often driven by fear and as such can impact on the enjoyment of the individual and their long-term participation in the sport.

Punishment in the form of criticism can decrease unwanted behaviours, but it can also have undesirable side effects, such as arousing the fear of failure, increasing anxiety, and causing obstacles to be viewed as threats rather than challenges. Those with a high fear of failure perform less well in competition, have a higher risk of injury, enjoy the sport less, and are more likely to drop out (Smith, 2001).

Punishment should not, however, be completely avoided. It is useful for situations involving breaches of the health and safety rules and other major disciplinary actions. When used sparingly, it can be used as a shock tactic to highlight the seriousness of a situation.

The use of feedback to reinforce a desired behaviour is the best way to eliminate mistakes. Rather than trying to stamp out errors using feedback such as "don't let your heels come up" or "don't tip forward", the correct behaviour can be reinforced by using comments such as "keep stretching your calf muscle down and think about growing tall". Feedback should always focus on improving rather than not making a mistake. This approach ensures that riders view mistakes as opportunities to learn, even if it is learning how not to do something!

Using positive reinforcement is more complicated than simply providing praise when something is done well. The coach needs to understand what type of positive reinforcement works for each individual rider. For example some riders like to be praised in front of the group, whilst others might be embarrassed to be singled out and do anything to avoid that happening.

In addition, the rider needs to understand why the reinforcement has been given so they can recreate the behaviour or action. This enables them to feel in control of their own performance. The coach must be specific about what they are praising.

If verbal praise is the main form of positive reinforcement, aim to vary the words that are used so it is not seen as a standard, automatic response. Combine this with an instructional reminder. For example, "well-ridden; you kept looking ahead and rode him forward into the contact."

Reinforcement also forces the coach to be clear in their own minds about exactly which behaviours they want to reinforce. Clearly, this is likely to depend on the progress and ability of each individual rider and the different stages in a rider's development (Smith, 2001).

Positive reinforcement can also be used to reinforce a rider's:

- Good sportsmanship
- Adherence to rules
- Teamwork
- Support and encouragement of others in the group
- Effort
- Consideration for the horse and its training

It is important not only to praise the rider who has performed well but also the rider who has tried and failed. Reinforce the effort as much as the results because this is what the rider has direct control over. If reinforcement is used to praise the ability of the horse or rider (rather than what the rider does), there can be a perceived lack of control, which may affect motivation since ability is something intangible; you either have it or you don't.

Receiving Feedback

The coach should also learn to read the non-verbal feedback of a rider. For instance fidgeting and turned-down eyes can indicate boredom or disinterest; fully raised eyebrows are a good indicator of disbelief, and frowning of puzzlement. At the same time as displaying these behaviours the rider may be saying, "yes, I understand". Clearly their non-verbal messages do not agree with their words, and further explanation may be needed.

It is also a skill to be able to receive verbal feedback whether from a rider, another coach, a mentor, or an assessor. A coach may not agree with the feedback, but they need to accept that it is the person's opinion based on what they've seen or how they feel. Regardless of the coach's own feelings, they must respect the other's viewpoint. Thank them for their input, be positive, and go away and think about what has been said before deciding if it is something that needs to be acted upon or not.

The Coach/Parent Relationship

Research by Stewart (1994) suggested that parents want coaches who are fair and honest in their dealings with the riders they are coaching. A coach should also be committed to the rider enjoying their riding and dedicated to the development of good sportsmanship. In fact, parents were most likely to rank the following last in terms of priority:

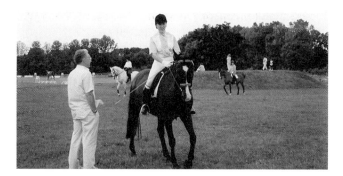

Figure 1.8 Coaches should be able to communicate effectively with the parents and relatives of those they coach, who often travel with the rider to coaching sessions and competitions.

- Commitment to winning
- Extensive personal experience as a rider
- Improving rider's chances of riding at a higher level

Much of the research indicated that there is often a discrepancy between what parents want and what coaches think parents want. Parents consistently ranked sportsmanship higher than coaches expected and competing at a higher level lower than coaches expected. This reinforces the need for coaches to possess strong communication skills so that they are able to correctly identify and interpret the messages being given by riders and their parents or other family members (Figure 1.8).

SUMMARY

- *Instructor*, *trainer*, and *coach* are all terms used to describe individuals involved in working with horses and riders. The general perception is that instructors aim to improve basic skills, trainers aim to improve the horse, and coaches work with elite level riders and teams.
- Four models of coaching have been identified: standard or traditional model, general educational model, humanistic model, and invitational model.
- A coach may be required to fulfil many roles and should develop their own coaching philosophy to ensure their goals and ambitions are not lost in those of the riders they are coaching.
- The main purpose of coaching is to develop the rider's physical and psychological skills in order for them to be able to ride safely and effectively.
- A coach's main responsibility is to the health and welfare of the horse and rider. Enjoyment, challenge, and improvement, rather than winning, should be the ideal outcomes.
- Coaches should be aware of and reflect on the impact of their expectations on riders.

- Coaching styles can be categorised as either coach-centred or rider-centred, depending on the coach's predominant approach.
- Effective coaching is determined by the nature of the problem or situation and the subsequent response of the coach rather than the inherent personality of the coach.
- Effective communication is fundamental to coaching, and consideration should be given to developing both verbal and non-verbal methods of communication as well as active listening skills.
- Feedback can have the single biggest impact on the quality of learning, so the quality, quantity, and strategy for providing feedback is important.
- Feedback can serve as reinforcement (positive or negative) or punishment. The aim is either to increase or decrease the likelihood of a behaviour being repeated.

Self Study

1. Observe a number of different coaches and identify
   - Their coaching style (rider-centred vs coach-centred)
   - How they communicate with riders (verbal and non-verbal)
   - Any potential barriers to communication
   - How they provide feedback to riders
   - Any feedback strategies they use

2. Comment on the appropriateness and success of the coach's approach.

Exam Style Questions

1. Discuss the appropriateness of the four coaching models identified by Lombardo in coaching different types of riders.
2. Explain why it is important for coaches to be aware of the expectations they have of the riders they coach.
3. Describe the key features of effective communication.
4. Differentiate between the methods of feedback available to the coach. Give examples.

REFERENCES

Chelladurai, P. and Saleh, S. (1980). Dimensions of leader behaviour in sports: Development of a leadership scale. *Journal of Sport Psychology*, 2, 34–45.

Chelladurai, P. and Trail, G. (2001). Styles of decision making in coaching. In *Applied Sport Psychology: Personal Growth to Peak Performance* (edited by J.M. Williams), 107–119. California: Mayfield Publishing Company.

Hardin, B. (1999). Expertise in teaching and coaching: A qualitative study of physical educators and athletic coaches. *Sociology of Sport Online*, Vol. 2, issue 1.

Housner, L.D. and Griffey, D.C. (1985). Teacher cognition: Differences in planning and interactive decision making between experienced and inexperienced teachers. *Research Quarterly for Exercise and Sport*, 56, 45–53.

Lombardo, B.J. (1999). Coaching in the 21st century: Issues, concerns and solutions. *Sociology of Sport Online*, Vol. 2, issue 1.

Lyle, J., Allison, M. and Taylor, J. (1997). *Factors Influencing the Motivations of Sport Coaches* – Research Report No.49, Edinburgh: The Scottish Sports Council.

Murray, M.C. and Mann, B.L. (2001). Leadership Effectiveness. In *Applied Sport Psychology: Personal Growth to Peak Performance* (edited by J.M. Williams), 82–106. California: Mayfield Publishing Company.

Pieron, M. and Goncalves, C. (1987). Participation engagement and teacher's feedback in physical education teaching and coaching. In *Myths, Models and Methods in Sport Pedagogy* (edited by M. Pieron), 249–254. Champaign, IL: Human Kinetics.

Smoll, F.L. and Smith, R.E. (2001) Conducting sport psychology training programs for coaches: Cognitive-behavioural principles and techniques. In *Applied Sport Psychology: Personal Growth to Peak Performance* (edited by J.M. Williams), 378–393. California: Mayfield Publishing Company.

Smith, R.E. (2001). Positive reinforcement, performance feedback and performance enhancement. In *Applied Sport Psychology: Personal Growth to Peak Performance* (edited by J.M. Williams), 29–42. California: Mayfield Publishing Company.

Smith, R.E. and Smoll, F.L. (1997). Coaching the coaches: Youth sports as a scientific and applied behavioural setting. *Current Directions in Psychological Science*, 6, 16–21.

Sports Coach UK (2004). *Sports Coaching in the UK*. Leeds: Sports Coach UK.

Sternberg Horn, T., Lox, C.L. and Labrador, F. (2001). The self-fulfilling prophecy theory: When Coaches' expectations become reality. In *Applied Sport Psychology: Personal Growth to Peak Performance* (edited by J.M. Williams), 63–81. California: Mayfield Publishing Company.

Stewart, C. (1994). Parents and coaches: Expectations, attitudes and communication. *Physical Educator*, 51, 130–136.

Valle, C.N. and Bloom, G.A. (2005). Building a successful university program: Key and common elements of expert coaches. *Journal of Applied Sport Psychology*. 17:3, 179–196.

Understanding the Individual

Chapter Objective

To provide an overview of the theories of motivation; guidelines on psychological skills for riders and recommendations for the setting of goals.

2.1 MOTIVATION

It is a commonly held belief that individuals are either motivated or they are not. In other words, motivation is something you are born with, and if not, you will need motivating by someone or something. The reality, as always, is more complex.

Most people are motivated to do things that are enjoyable or at which they are successful. The challenge for riders and coaches alike is how to keep motivated when things are not going well, for instance, when training gets hard and repetitive, progress is slow, or the horse or rider is injured.

Duda and Treasure (2001) discovered that in sport, motivation is strengthened when individuals feel competent and in control of their performance. This sense of control and competence can be influenced, both positively and negatively, in four key areas.

- Self-efficacy (commonly referred to as self-confidence)
- Attributions

- Motivation orientation
- Achievement motivation

Self-Efficacy

Self-efficacy is an individual's belief in their ability to perform a task successfully. Those with high levels of self-efficacy will try harder and persist longer, whereas those with low self-efficacy tend to experience greater levels of anxiety and give up when things get difficult.

There are many strategies available to coaches to increase a rider's self-efficacy. The most effective ones include providing opportunities for the riders to feel successful. This involves praising the completion of training exercises and encouraging riders to take pride and satisfaction in past successes. A lack of success should be seen positively as an opportunity to learn rather than as a failure. Goal setting, modelling, and positive self talk are also highly effective (Bandura, 1997).

Terminology

Modelling is when individuals imagine themselves to have the characteristics of someone they respect or admire. For instance a rider may consider John Whitaker to be the epitome of self-confidence, and so they will try to think and act like John Whitaker in order to improve their own levels of self-confidence.

Watching others perform successfully is especially effective in increasing levels of confidence in younger riders or those with limited experience. It may involve watching someone complete a dressage test or a round of show jumping or it may be seeing someone of similar ability and experience execute a three-loop serpentine. The underlying principle is "they can do it, so can I". However, care should be taken to avoid this becoming a competitive situation rather than an educational one.

Watching other riders and modelling their actions and behaviours can help increase confidence. If an individual is feeling nervous or anxious about a competition, imagining how someone respected and admired would act and attempting to think, behave, and ride like them can help. Sometimes it is worth asking the question, "What would Michael Whitaker, Pippa Funnell, or Richard Davison do in this situation?"

Remembering or watching previous good performances or successful completions of a test, course, or type of jump can be a useful source of self-confidence. A rider gains confidence by knowing that they have done something before and therefore can do it again. Often the temptation is to watch replays of things that have gone wrong to analyse why and how. This constant reliving or replaying of mistakes can seriously damage an individual's self-confidence. Instead, energy should be devoted to analysing why things went well and how that performance can be replicated (Figure 2.1a–d).

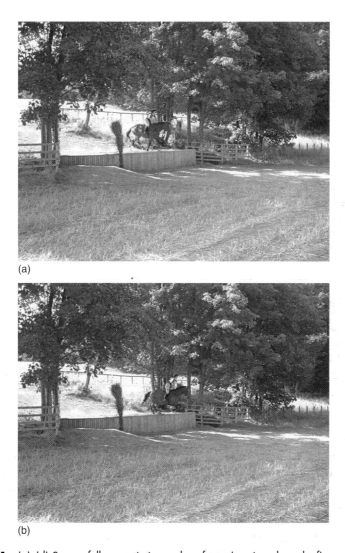

(a)

(b)

Figure 2.1   (a)–(d) Successfully negotiating a drop fence (continued overleaf).

The final element to increasing confidence levels is self talk. Positive self talk helps individuals focus on their performance, stay in the present, and maintain their concentration levels. It is particularly important for coaches to consider this area as it may be what riders are saying to themselves that limits their performance. For example, a rider who, despite all the encouragement from their coach goes into the start box saying to themselves, "I know I'm going to mess this up", will, more often than not, encounter problems.

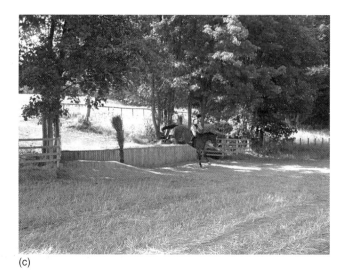

(c)

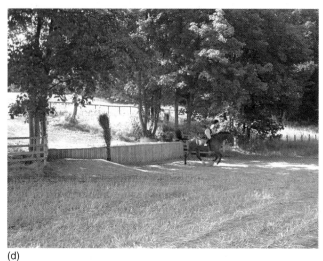

(d)

Figure 2.1 *Continued*

Case Study 2.1

Sam is a keen eventer who has just started competing at Intro level. She has been coached by Lorna for six months and found that the sessions have boosted her confidence and improved her riding. However, when she gets to a competition she often rides well below her ability. Lorna suggests a number of key words for Sam to remember and repeat to herself during each phase.

For the dressage Lorna suggests that Sam repeat to herself "smile", as this seems to help her relax and subsequently so does her horse.

In the show jumping Sam has a tendency to override into the fences, and this often results in a few knock-downs as her horse stands off or puts in an extra stride. By repeating to herself "wait" on the approach to each fence, Sam sits quieter and allows her horse to jump more correctly.

Cross country is their strongest phase, but when the fences are less straight-forward Sam tends to look down and often ends up in front of the movement. To combat this Lorna advises her to tell herself to "look up" on the approach to each fence.

Simple Exercise for Demonstrating Power of Self Talk

Ask the riders to stand with one arm stretched out sideways at shoulder height. Ask another rider to push down on the outstretched arm.

As their arms are being pushed down, ask them to repeat the words "strong and powerful, strong and powerful" over and over, ideally aloud.

Now try the same exercise again with the riders repeating over and over "weak and feeble, weak and feeble".

Both groups of riders should notice the difference. When the words, "strong and powerful" are being repeated, it is much more difficult to push the arm down. When a rider is repeating weak and feeble, the arm can be pushed down much more easily.

Being able to recognise and manage a rider's emotional and psychological state is an important skill, particularly for those aiming to offer competition coaching. Some riders view competition nerves as helping their performance, allowing them to get up for the competition. Other riders view nerves as detrimental to their per-formance, causing tension and poor riding. Relaxation exercises can help the rider to relax and reduce nerves. Loud, energetic music or movement can be used to help the rider who feels they need to increase their energy levels before a competition (Figure 2.2 and 2.3).

Attributions

Attributions are the reasons an individual gives to explain why something hap-pened. They usually fall into four categories skill or ability, effort, task difficulty, and luck (Table 2.1).

The attributions a rider makes for their success or failure is important as it affects their motivation levels and their future expectations of success and failure. Knowing a rider's attributions can help coaches understand:

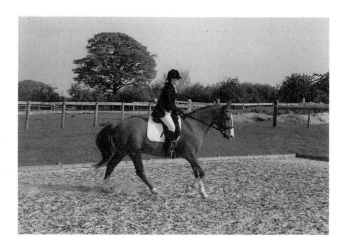

Figure 2.2 Horse and rider look tense and lacking confidence.

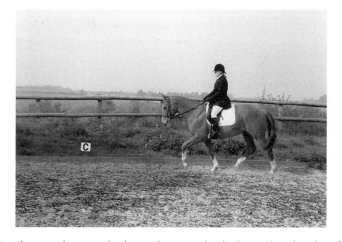

Figure 2.3 The same horse and rider on the same day looking relaxed and confident.

Table 2.1. Attributions.

	Reasons for Success	**Reasons for Failure**
Ability/skill	I rode well today	I rode like a sack of potatoes.
Effort	I've worked hard to improve my fitness	I was a bit lazy in my preparation today.
Task difficulty	Cross country is my best phase	I can't ride related distances.
Luck	I was lucky to be drawn last	I was unlucky to roll a pole.

- How to keep a rider motivated.
- What expectations a rider has about their own and other's abilities.
- How to help the rider improve their performance.
- How a rider can feel satisfied with their performance.

The way a rider explains their performance provides the coach with key information about the level of control and influence they feel they have over it. A person who takes sole responsibility for their performance, win or lose, is considered to have an internal locus of control. The rider who puts good and bad performances down to factors outside of their control is considered to have an external locus of control.

Internal Locus of Control

Individuals who have an internal locus of control believe that what they do influences the result they get. They will often explain their performances in terms of the effort they put in and the skills they have. Attributing outcomes to their own efforts creates emotions such as pride, "my preparation paid off", and shame, "I've let people down". This internalising of success can lead to increased self-confidence (Figure 2.4). In contrast, internalising failure can lead to feelings of incompetence and eventual withdrawal from the sport.

External Locus of Control

Individuals who have an external locus of control believe outcomes are influenced by external factors such as luck, fate, other people (e.g., judges), or their horses. When successful, these riders tend to believe they have had little influence over the outcome and as a result can become de-motivated and lose interest in the sport. Attributing failure to external factors can lead to frustration and anger as the rider feels powerless to do anything to change the outcome in the future.

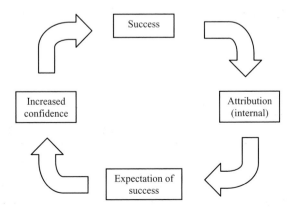

Figure 2.4   Positive confidence cycle.

Coaches need to be aware of the reasons *they* attribute to a rider's successes and failures. To increase feelings of control and competence the rider needs to be encouraged to view success as something that is within their control and unlikely to change. Lack of success should be viewed as likely to change and is within the rider's control to change in the future (Weiner, 1986).

When a coach attributes an error or below expected performance to lack of effort, lack of practice, or some other rider-controlled factor, it helps to facilitate future motivation. It also helps to prevent against feelings of helplessness and encourages a positive attitude (Steinberg Horn et al, 2001).

Motivation Orientation

The attribution theory of motivation considers the reasons riders give for their performances. The orientation theory of motivation considers what motivates riders to participate in riding in the first place. Generally, this falls into two categories: intrinsic motivation and extrinsic motivation (Figure 2.5).

Intrinsically motivated riders have an innate need to feel competent and self-determining, that is, in control. They will participate in an activity without receiving any apparent reward because they find the activity itself rewarding. In effect they motivate themselves internally. An individual who is intrinsically motivated is referred to as having a task orientation. It is desirable to encourage riders to be intrinsically motivated as this is likely to ensure their long-term participation in the sport and lead to greater resilience when things are not going well.

Extrinsically motivated riders have an innate need to be recognised and will participate in an activity for the rewards or status it offers. In effect, they are motivated by the external benefits on offer. An individual who is extrinsically motivated is often referred to as having an ego orientation. Having an ego orientation is a powerful motivator when things are going well but is poor at sustaining motivation when the inevitable slumps in performance occur. This is because the individuals are drawing their confidence and self-worth from factors that are not wholly within their control. Table 2.2 details the characteristics of task-oriented and ego-oriented individuals.

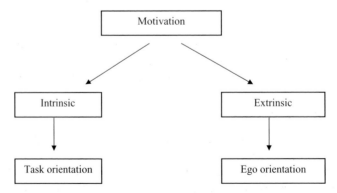

Figure 2.5   Motivation orientation.

Table 2.2. Task orientation and ego orientation characteristics.

Task Oriented	Ego Oriented
Focus on self	Focus on others
Comparison to own previous performances	Comparison to other's performance
Focus energy on fulfilment of task	Concerned with achieving more than others
Goal directed:	Outcome oriented:
Executing a piaffe to passage transition	Qualifying for horse of the year show
Completing Badminton	Being appointed captain
Completing a 25-mile endurance ride	Getting a sponsorship deal
Learning a new skill	Winning the most prize money
Doing one's very best	Scoring the highest percentage
Training a horse to medium level	Going up in ranking
Turning out a horse well	Winning by large margin
Riding at Hickstead	Being picked for the team
Feelings of competence not constrained by others	Feelings of competence controlled by the performance of others
Believes everyone can demonstrate ability through effort and improvement	Believes only one person can be the best
Increased persistence, effort, and interest in challenging tasks regardless of how competent he or she feels	Likely to give up and lose interest if failure is likely
Believe sport should teach the value of trying one's best, cooperating with others, following the rules, and being a good sport	Believe sport is about winning
Place emphasis on skills mastery	Emphasis is on achieving more than others
Main purpose of sport is to gain skill/ knowledge, to exhibit effort, to perform at one's best, and to experience personal improvement	View sport as a means to an end, for example, popularity/wealth/celebrity

Source: Duda (1989)

Coaches can use positive reinforcement to promote intrinsic motivation with statements such as, "great job", "you ought to feel proud of yourself for that effort", "you've really mastered that exercise", "that was a big improvement on last year's performance", "your hard work has really paid off", and "you both looked like you enjoyed that". Emphasising the intrinsic challenge, personal satisfaction, and sources of enjoyment helps to take the mind off the extrinsic rewards.

Achievement Motivation

Some riders are motivated to achieve success. These individuals like to be evaluated, value feedback from others, look for challenges, and are not afraid of failure. Others are driven to succeed because they have a deep-rooted fear of failure. These riders tend to avoid challenges, are preoccupied with failure and perform poorly when evaluated.

If the probability of success is high, the need to achieve is weakened because the reward for success is low, that is, it is expected. If the probability of success is low and failure is likely, the need to avoid failure is weakened because the reward for success is high, that is, it is unexpected. This explains why a rider who is focused on avoiding failure will often choose tasks that are either very simple and success is virtually guaranteed or tasks that are very difficult where it is highly likely that they will fail.

Self-motivation is an aspect of achievement motivation. It is the extent to which a person will persist in a task. It is closely related to intrinsic motivation but refers to riders who keep going on a task when the task itself is not immediately motivating, such as fitness training, cleaning tack, mucking out, etc.

Individuals also use goals to evaluate an experience as a success or a failure. The goals that are set should be performance oriented (within the riders control) rather than outcome oriented (winning). Goals that focus on gains in skills and knowledge, effort levels, and self determined criteria for success are more likely to increase intrinsic motivation.

Success should not be seen in terms of winning. Success must be seen in terms of riders exceeding their own goals rather than surpassing the performance of others. If a coach encourages individuals to understand and implement this principle, they will have done more to help them become excellent riders and successful adults than by any other coaching action.

2.2   GOAL ACHIEVEMENT

Goal setting is the process by which an individual plans what they are trying to accomplish. Goals focus the rider's attention on what is important; they provide a purpose for their efforts, maintain motivation, help to organise training, and increase confidence by highlighting progress and improvement. Research has shown that goal setting clearly and consistently facilitates improved performance (Locke and Latham, 1985).

Riders may have short-, intermediate-, or long-term goals (Table 2.3), and these may be performance, process, or outcome oriented (Table 2.4).

There is a commonly held belief that all goals should be realistic, flexible, and within a time frame. However, this varies depending on the type of goal. Longer-term aims and goals (LTAs and LTGs) are unlikely to be as powerful or as motivating if they keep changing or if they lack the challenge of having to push oneself to achieve them. Equally, if goals have too rigid a time frame, they can be demotivating and set the rider up to fail.

Obviously, if a rider's LTA is to compete at the 2012 London Olympics, then this is a fixed and unchanging time frame. However, if their LTA is to ride in top hat and tails, the actual date this is achieved can be flexible. Short-term goals should be given the highest priority because through achieving these, progress will be made towards the intermediate- and long-term targets.

Outcome goals are often important for those involved in competitions. However, since they are rarely within the total control of the rider, they should be supported

Table 2.3.   Timetable of goals.

Long-term aim (LTA)	This is the big goal. What the rider wants to achieve in the long term, for example, Olympic medal, team selection, competing in top hat and tails.
Long-term goals (LTG)	The long-term aim may be made up of several long-term goals. These goals are the stepping stones to achieving the long-term aim, for example, complete Badminton, ride at Grand Prix level, qualify for National Championships.
Intermediate-term goals (ITG)	These are the goals to be accomplished in a shorter time frame and may be related to a specific competition or things to be achieved each month or by the end of the season. They should help the progression towards achieving the long-term goals and can comprise training, skill, fitness, psychological, or competition goals to ensure the rider is on target for their LTG.
Short-term goals (STG)	These are the goals used to set daily or weekly targets and should be short and specific. They provide feedback about progress and should help to achieve the intermediate goals. To keep the rider motivated they must provide small, regular experiences of success, which enhance motivation.

Table 2.4.   Types of goals.

Performance goals	These goals are specific to the rider and their performance, or if the rider has more than one horse or competes in more than one discipline they would be specific for that horse and rider combination. These goals might relate to improving personal best scores or improving compared to previous performances.
Outcome goals	These generally relate to winning or beating another rider. They are less effective than performance goals as the rider often has only partial control over the result since the ability and form of the opponents can be influencing factors. Focusing purely on the result can increase anxiety and reduce confidence and motivation.
Process goals	These goals relate to the actions or techniques that are required to achieve success. For instance a rider who has a tendency to become overly concerned with the results of other competitors might set a goal to look only at his or her own scores.

Source: Martens (1987) and Hardy et al (1996)

by performance goals. For instance, a rider may have the goal of winning a dressage qualifier. To do this they believe they will need to score over 70%. This is their performance goal. Process goals should identify what areas are within a riders control and will contribute to achieving such a score. These might include riding forward in all the transitions, ensuring each movement is started and finished at the appropriate marker, or staying relaxed and focused throughout the test.

Pierce and Burton (1998) suggest that individuals who set performance goals are more likely to adopt a problem solving approach to competition. They rarely perceive unsuccessful results as failure; instead, they develop strategies to over-come difficulties and demonstrate tremendous persistence in the face of adversity.

Clearly, goals are not restricted to competitive riders. A beginner or novice may want to set a goal to be able to complete a round of show jumps or to ride a dres-sage test. Some riders may decide that in order to improve their riding, they need to get fitter, lose weight, or develop their strength and flexibility, and goals can help them achieve this. The fundamental principle behind goal setting is for the coach and rider to assess where they are currently, where they want to be and what steps need to be taken to close the gap between the two.

Case Study 2.2

Subject: Female event rider
Standard: BE Intro level

Goal-Setting Plan – Long and Intermediate Term Goals

Long-term aim	Complete Scottish Open Championships CIC***
Long-term goal	Get CIC** qualifying result (qualifying result = less than 50 penalties dressage, maximum 16 penalties show jumping; maximum 20 jump penalties, and maximum 36 time penalties cross country)
Long-term goal	Get qualifying result at Advanced (qualifying result as above)
Intermediate goal	Five clears cross country at Intermediate level
Intermediate goal	Complete Scottish Novice Championships
Intermediate goal	Two clears cross country at Intermediate level
Intermediate goal	Top three finish at Novice level
Intermediate goal	Five clears cross country at Novice level
Intermediate goal	Five clears cross country at Pre-Novice level
Intermediate goal	Five clears cross country at Intro level

Goal-Setting Plan – Intermediate and Short Term Goals

Intermediate goal	Five clears cross country at Intro level	By end 2007
Short-term goal	Complete Beamish Intro with clear cross country	Oct 2007
Short-term goal	Complete Hunwick Intro with clear cross country	Aug 2007
Short-term goal	Complete Hendersyde Intro with clear cross country	Aug 2007
Short-term goal	Complete Cumwhinton Intro with clear cross country	July 2007
Short-term goal	Complete Hexham Intro with clear cross country	June 2007
Short-term goal	Complete Ivesley Intro	April 2007
Short-term goal	Two dressage and one show jumping training session One cross country training session	March 2007
Short-term goal	Fitness work 3–4 days at walk, trot, and canter Two to three days of schooling (flat and jump)	Feb 2007
Short-term goal	Fitness work three to four days, add canter intervals Introduce schooling one to two days	Week 4 2007
Short-term goal	Fitness work 60–90 minutes, five days per week	Week 3 2007
Short-term goal	Fitness work 30–60 minutes, four days per week	Week 2 2007
Short-term goal	Fitness work 20–30 minutes, three days per week, walk and trot	Week 1 2007

The time scales on these short-term goals should be flexible so that if the horse or rider is injured, they can be adjusted. Equally, they may need to be amended if, for instance, a problem occurs in the cross country phase and it is necessary to take a break from competition until the problem is resolved.

Goal Evaluation

Goal	Fitness work 20–30 minutes, three days per week, walk and trot
Completed by	7th Jan 2007
Outcome	Achieved
Evaluation	Difficult, as the weather and going has not been good. Horse has coped well and ready to progress.

It is important to evaluate each goal individually at the end of the time frame to allow for any adjustments to the plan to be made. In this case if the weather had prevented the rider from completing the fitness work the time frame would need to be extended and this has a knock-on effect for subsequent goals.

Guidelines on goal setting for coaches are as follows:

- Ensure that riders set goals that are specific and measurable. This means having goals that they will recognise when they've achieved them. "To do your best" is an admirable goal, but what exactly does it mean to actually do your best? A better goal might be to be able to consistently score above 60% by the end of the season or increase their personal best score to 75%.
- Riders should set goals that are moderately difficult but realistic so that they are both challenging and achievable.
- There should be short-term as well as long-term goals. Most riders who set goals will have long-term aspirations. However, short-term goals allow immediate improvements in performance to be seen and therefore increase motivation and confidence.
- Goal setting should include process, performance, and outcome goals. Research has shown that this is most likely to facilitate the achievement of long-term goals.
- Riders should have goals for training and competition
- Target dates for achievement of goals should be included, especially for short- and intermediate-term goals.
- The rider should identify strategies for achieving the goals. For instance a show jumper who has set themselves the goal of consistently jumping double clears over the summer season must identify what they need to do in order to achieve this goal. It might mean doing an extra schooling session on the flat each week or taking more time to set the horse up before each jump.
- Goals should be written down and kept visible. This helps keep training and competition focused.
- Ensure adequate time is spent on evaluation. Feedback is critical if goals are to enhance performance.

(Gould, 2001)

Performance Profiling

In sports, which tend to concentrate on outcomes (win or lose), it can often be difficult for riders to engage with other types of goals. Performance profiling is a useful technique for identifying process goals for training and competition that are both motivating and engaging. It is also a good opportunity for the coach and rider to identify and openly discuss areas in need of improvement (Dale and Wrisberg, 1996).

There are two approaches, the first requires the rider to identify someone they admire, aspire to be like, or view as particularly successful. A list is made of the characteristics they consider fundamental to this persons success and score themselves against each individually. This provides the coach with an insight into how the rider views their own skills and abilities and what aspects they consider important to good performance (Butler and Hardy, 1992). Table 2.5 illustrates this approach. (A blank profile is included in the appendices.)

Alternatively, the rider is asked to consider their long term aim and identify the qualities they feel are needed to achieve it. Each quality is then rated according to its importance and the rider awards themselves a score for each based on their current performance (Table 2.6).

From this information, goals can be developed to bridge the gap between where the rider feels they are today and where they would like to be. For instance, the

Table 2.5. Performance profiling 1.

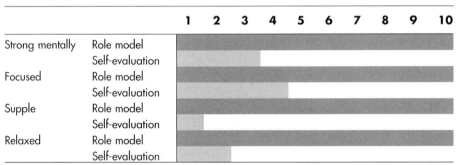

Table 2.6. Performance profiling 2.

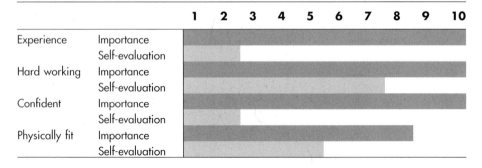

rider who views relaxation as a desirable characteristic might set a goal to practice relaxation techniques for 15 minutes every day. The rider who believes that experience and confidence is necessary to achieve their long-term aim may set themselves the goal of doing more competitions at a lower level or riding a school master to gain confidence.

2.3   PSYCHOLOGICAL SKILLS

Personality

Researchers have studied personality for years in an attempt to predict winners, identify the right personality for a particular sport, and differentiate between the personality characteristics of elite and novice performers. Although there is little evidence to suggest a link between sporting performance and personality, for the sake of completeness Table 2.7 provides a brief summary of the main theories.

Table 2.7. Theories of personality.

Body type	Believes a person's physique predicts his or her personality and can be catagorised into three distinct types: • Ectomorphs are thin, lean individuals who are shy, introverted, and inhibited. • Endomorphs are typically rounder and more prone to fat. They are outgoing, confident, and warm. • Mesomorphs are more muscular, have an adventurous spirit, and can be prone to aggression.
Trait theory	Believes an individual can be classified as either extrovert or introvert, stable or unstable, and that they will always react according to those traits whatever the situation. • Extroverts seek change and excitement, become bored easily, and are poor at tasks requiring concentration. • Introverts prefer calm and quiet, dislike the unexpected, and are good at tasks requiring concentration. • Stable individuals are even tempered, emotionally stable, and easy going. • Unstable individuals are restless, excitable, and anxious.
Social learning theory	Suggests that personality and behaviour is determined by the environment and experiences an individual has as they grow up. Personality is not inherited but is formed as a result of upbringing.
Interactionist theory	Combines both social learning and trait theory by suggesting that certain personality characteristics can predict behaviour in some, but not all, situations. For example, a rider does not normally experience anxiety, but does become anxious when competing. This concept is known as the trait/state theory. A trait is something that is exhibited normally in most situations, and a state is something that is only exhibited in certain situations.

Source: Gill (2000)

Attention and Concentration

Attention and concentration are terms that are often used interchangeably and refer to the ability to selectively focus on some things while disregarding others. This ability can have a profound influence on performance. In essence the brain is unable to look at two different things or think two different thoughts at exactly the same time which is why practice is so important. Practicing a skill enables an individual to perform it automatically thus leaving the brain free to focus and react to the external environment. It is also why imagery and positive self talk are key to successful performance (Figures 2.6 and 2.7).

Riders are likely to have a preferred concentration style. They may tend to focus on their own thoughts and feelings or on external objects and events. However,

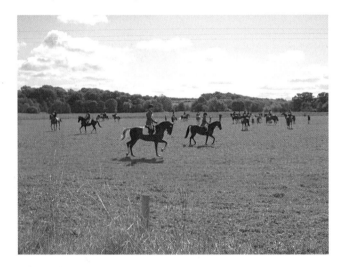

Figure 2.6 A busy dressage warm-up area.

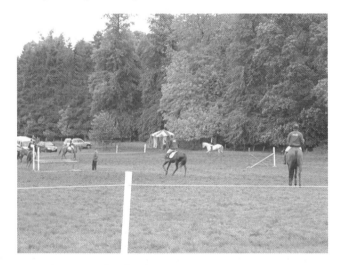

Figure 2.7 Lots to be aware of in the show jumping warm up.

different types of concentration are required for different tasks and disciplines, so riders should be able to adapt their style according to the requirements of the situation.

Concentration has two dimensions, broad or narrow and internal or external (Table 2.8 and Figure 2.8). Broad refers to an individual's ability to focus on

Table 2.8. Types of concentration.

Broad/External	Used to assess situations by taking in large amounts of information	Polo Handball Racing
Broad/Internal	Ideal for analysing performances and planning strategies	Coach Team manager Team captain All disciplines
Narrow/External	Ability to act and react to what is going on; requiring focus on an object in the external environment	Show jumping Cross country
Narrow/Internal	Ideal for learning new skills, mental rehearsal, and focusing on own riding and how the horse is going	Dressage Endurance

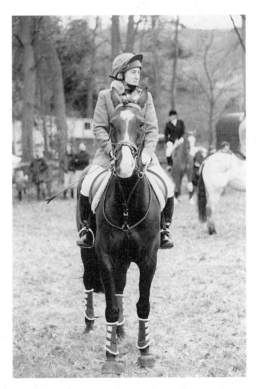

Figure 2.8 A picture of concentration at a day's drag hunting. The rider is demonstrating a broad external focus, watching for the signal to head off. The horse is demonstrating a narrow external focus, alert for the signal from the rider to start moving.

information from different sources. Narrow is the ability to ignore distractions and focus on a specific thing. Internal is when the rider's concentration is focused on their own thoughts and feelings and external concentration is when the rider focuses on what is happening around them (Nideffer and Sagal, 2001).

The coach can use this knowledge to direct the rider's attention in the most appropriate direction.

Case Study 2.3

Adam runs monthly all-day coaching sessions for event riders. This month the morning session is concentrating on flatwork and test riding, the afternoon focuses on grid work and riding a course of show jumps, followed by a session on walking cross country courses.

During the flatwork session Adam asks the riders to initially focus on different parts of their body whilst warming up. *Narrow/internal*

Working systematically from the head down, the riders are asked to pay attention to:

- Where they are looking
- The position of their shoulders
- The position of their hands
- The weight in the reins
- The movement in their seat
- The contact of their legs with the horse
- The flexibility in their ankles

The riders are asked to then focus their attention on the horse. *Narrow/external*

- The activity of the hind legs
- The evenness of stride length
- The rhythm of the steps
- The swinging of the back
- The lift of the shoulders
- The contact with the bit
- The expression of the ears

When practising riding the tests, riders are asked to broaden their focus to formulate a plan about how they are going to use the arena to set up each movement and where they are going to perform transitions and half halts. *Broad/internal*

The show jumping session starts with grid work and riders are asked to focus on what is happening on the approach and over the fences. Firstly they are asked to focus on themselves. *Narrow/internal*

- Where they are looking
- The position of the upper body

- The position of the lower leg
- The position and movement of the hands

Then they are asked to focus on the horse. *Narrow/external*

- Straightness
- Speed
- Impulsion
- Technique

The group now moves on to jumping a course. Again the riders are asked to broaden their focus to include the types of jumps, the going and the approaches to each fence. The riders each take it in turn to jump the course, and Andrew then identifies one thing for each person that he would like them to focus on next time. *Broad/internal*

One rider is asked to focus on a point beyond each jump to ensure they keep straight and upright in their upper body. Another is asked to focus on the rhythm of the horse's canter to promote balance and control. The third rider is asked to focus on waiting for the fence to encourage her to sit still rather than chasing the horse into each jump. For the final rider, Andrew places several cones around the course and asks the rider to focus on going round the cones to improve the approach to the fences.

The final session involves Andrew and the group walking a cross country course. On the first walk round the group are encouraged to take a *broad, external focus* by paying attention to the ground conditions, siting of the fences, positioning of flags, alternative routes, and any potential hazards (Figure 2.9).

On the second walk, the riders are asked to take a *broad, internal focus* to plan how they are going to ride the course, taking into consideration the approach to the fence, their route through the obstacle, where they are going to jump each fence, the options if they have a problem, and where they can make up time.

On their third walk the riders are asked to switch to a *narrow, internal focus* of attention to mentally rehearse their approach. The riders are encouraged to walk exactly where they are going to ride and rehearse in their minds exactly what they are going to do at each fence (Figures 2.10 and 2.11).

Stress and anxiety can alter the ways in which a rider is able to concentrate. There is a narrowing and internalising of attention resulting in the rider becoming preoccupied with worrying and limiting their ability to alter their focus. This can cause them to miss important external cues such as the bell going at the start of a show jumping round.

Arousal, Anxiety, and Stress

Stress is usually talked about in negative terms. People are often heard complaining about being stressed at work, during studying or when competing. However, stress

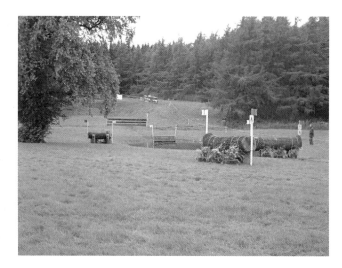

Figure 2.9   Being able to assess the ground conditions, siting, and alternative routes requires a broad, external focus.

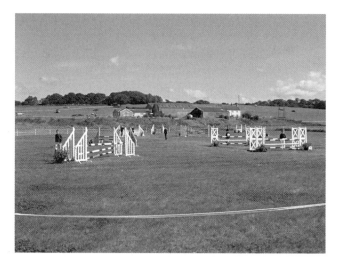

Figure 2.10   Being able to assess how to ride a show jumping course as a whole requires a broad, internal focus.

should not be seen as entirely negative. It provides the mental and physical energy needed to motivate us to do things and to do things well. Without an element of stress in our lives, we would become bored and psychologically stale.

Symptoms of too much stress can be physical (somatic), psychological (cognitive), or behavioural (Table 2.9). Somatic symptoms include racing heart, feelings of nausea, increased breathing rate, and sweating. Cognitive symptoms include worry, feelings of nervousness, and negative thoughts and images.

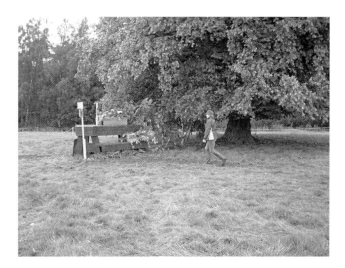

Figure 2.11 Walking the approach to a cross country fence requires a narrow, internal focus.

Table 2.9. Stress symptoms.

Physical	Psychological	Behavioural
Increased heart rate	Worry	Talking rapidly
Increased sweating	Feeling overwhelmed	Nail biting
Increased breathing rate	Inability to make decisions	Pacing
Dry mouth	Inability to concentrate	Yawning
Butterflies	Feeling out of control	Trembling
Nausea	Negative thoughts and images	Frequent trips to the toilet

Source: Davis et al (2005)

The terms arousal and anxiety are used to differentiate between the types of stress that a rider can experience. Arousal is considered to be the positive aspect of stress. The more aroused a rider is, the more interested and excited they are about a situation. Anxiety is considered to be the negative aspect of stress and can cause riders to "choke" during competition.

Arousal and Performance

There are four main theories to explain how arousal affects performance.

- Drive theory: Drive theory suggests that as arousal levels rise, so too does performance levels. However, this is only true for well-learnt skills. Beginners or novices do not benefit from increases in arousal during the early stages of learning. Equally complex skills can be inhibited by too high a level of arousal.

- Inverted U theory: This theory recognises that arousal does increase performance, but only up to a certain level. Once that optimum level of arousal has been reached, any further increase is actually detrimental and performance begins to decline.
- Catastrophe theory: This theory took the inverted U theory one step further and suggested that actually once the optimum level of arousal has been reached, any further increase in arousal leads to a catastrophic drop in performance, that is, choking.
- Zone of optimal functioning: This suggests that each individual has an optimum level of arousal for optimum performance. In equine sports, it is also necessary to consider the discipline in order to assess the affect of arousal. For instance, disciplines that require an attacking style of riding (polo, cross country, horseball) with high energy levels are likely to benefit from increased arousal. Those disciplines that require high levels of coordination and subtle movements (dressage, vaulting, reining) are likely to require much lower levels of arousal.

(Williams and Harris, 2001)

Anxiety and Performance

Individuals are often classified as either experiencing trait or state anxiety. Someone who has a predisposition to be anxious in a wide variety of situations and in all areas of their life exhibits trait anxiety. An individual who experiences a temporary negative stress reaction in certain situations is considered to exhibit state anxiety.

Competitive state anxiety is a temporary stress reaction to a competition, which can manifest in psychological, physiological, or behavioural symptoms. However, the effect on performance is likely to vary between riders, depending on whether they view "nerves" as helpful or not. Some riders relish the stress caused by competing and find that it brings out the best in them; others find it debilitating (Carver and Scheier, 1988).

Interestingly, other research has shown that it is the type of anxiety that is experienced that predicts the effect it will have on performance (Table 2.10). In general, cognitive anxiety is more likely to have a negative affect on performance than somatic anxiety, which appears to have a positive impact on performance (Martens et al, 1990).

Jones and Swain (1995) found that elite performers were more likely than non-elite performers to interpret any competitive anxiety as facilitating successful performance. Those who believed that anxiety limited their ability to perform tended to experience higher levels of cognitive anxiety.

Table 2.10. Types of anxiety.

Cognitive Anxiety	Somatic Anxiety
Increases during the days before a competition	Rises quickly a few hours before a competition
Fluctuates during performance	Tends to decrease during the competition

There are three main causes of competitive anxiety. The first is the nature of competition itself, in that there will be winners and losers. The second is the rider's concern about what other people will think, what they feel is expected of them and what they feel they owe others. The third is the pressure the rider puts on themselves by the way they talk to themselves (Rotella, 1983).

The role of the coach is to help the rider manage their levels of anxiety. This is achieved by riders being able to identify and maintain a level of arousal appropriate to their discipline and learning to view the symptoms of anxiety as positive to performance. Research has also shown that high levels of self-confidence act as a buffer to cognitive anxiety. The more a coach can do to promote the rider's self-confidence, the less likely they are to suffer the effects of cognitive anxiety (Hardy, 1996).

Psychological Skills Training

Research suggests that successful riders have better concentration, higher levels of self confidence, lower levels of anxiety and generally show more positive thoughts and determination than less successful riders (Gould and Weinberg, 1995; Meyers et al, 1999).

Therefore, developing a rider's mental skills is as important as developing their physical ones and as such requires a specifically designed training programme. Psychological skills training should be approached in the same way as any other training and include regular practice of at least 10–15 minutes per day, three to five days per week (Gould et al, 1990).

Psychological skills can be divided into three categories: those required for training, those required prior to the start of competition and those used during actual performance (Table 2.11).

However, before a coach decides to implement this type of training programme, they should practice the techniques themselves, ideally systematically and over a prolonged period of time. Personal experience is an essential ingredient in the ability to coach others through exercises and answer any questions that might arise. It is also important to lead by example as there is still considerable resistance to psychological training and it is often regarded as only for those who "have a problem". In fact, these types of techniques are valuable life skills that aim to develop individuals who are calm, confident and in control, whatever the situation (Weinberg and Williams, 2001).

Table 2.11. Psychological skills.

Training	Goal setting
	Motivation
Pre-competition	Mental imagery
	Self talk
During performance	Concentration
	Managing stress and anxiety

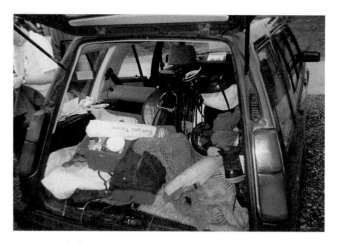

Figure 2.12   Organised chaos!

Riders and coaches should take the time to experiment with several of the following techniques in order to find the most effective strategies and develop individualised performance routines (Boutcher and Rotella, 1987).

Managing Stress and Anxiety: Preparation

Preparation is a key element to reducing stress. A rider should never attempt something in competition that they have not already succeeded in doing at home. Preparation also involves having everything ready that will be needed on competition day. Making a list of tack, grooming equipment, clothing, and all the show necessities helps to increase confidence by the knowledge that everything that will be needed has been accounted for. This ensures the rider can fully concentrate on their riding and not whether they remembered to pack an essential item of tack or equipment (Figure 2.12).

Taking time to plan the journey to the competition and allowing plenty of time for delays, finding the secretary on arrival and warming up is essential. Try to establish a routine at competitions. Riders should identify what needs to be done when they arrive, when they are going to get ready, when they are going to get the horse ready, when there is time for a tea break, how long they are going to warm up for, and what they are going to do in the warm-up. The more organised and planned a rider is the more control they will have over their stress levels.

A suitable backup plan is also an important part of being prepared. Once all possible outcomes have been considered and a suitable backup plan decided for each eventuality, the rider can relax and go back to thinking positive thoughts about a successful outcome.

Managing Stress and Anxiety: Relaxation

In order to relax, an individual needs to ensure they are breathing properly. A rider who is anxious or tense will tend to either hold their breath or breathe rapidly and shallowly from the upper chest. Learning to take a deep, slow, complete breath will usually trigger a relaxation response. A well-timed breath can provide the momentary relaxation required prior to entering the dressage arena or setting off cross country. There are many different breathing exercises, and riders should be encouraged to experiment to find the one that is most effective for them (Table 2.12).

Another relaxation technique is progressive muscular relaxation. This works on the principle that an anxious mind cannot exist when the body is relaxed, so it involves tensing and then relaxing muscles in a systematic way.

A rider should start at the face and work down the body, tensing each muscle for 5–10 seconds and then relaxing it. This also helps to develop awareness in the rider about what a tensed muscle feels like and what a relaxed muscle feels like in order to be better able to identify tension in their body. It is particularly common for riders to become tense in the neck and shoulder areas, so once they have learnt to spot tension, they can check these areas and roll the neck or shrug the shoulders to release it.

Table 2.12. Breathing exercises.

Complete breathing	With each breath, the rider should concentrate on the movement of the diaphragm. During inhalation, the diaphragm moves down, creating a vacuum and drawing in air. This forces the abdomen out, the chest to expand, and the rib cage to rise. The rider should hold the breath for a few seconds and then exhale by pulling the abdomen in and lowering the chest and shoulders to force the air out. At the end of the exhalation, the rider should let go of all muscular action so the abdomen and chest are completely relaxed.
Sighing	Sighing can help reduce tension. The rider should inhale slowly and hold the breath for 10 seconds, feeling the tension build in the throat and chest. The rider should exhale through the mouth with a slight sigh, letting all the tension leave the body with the breath. The idea is to focus in on the stillness after the sigh and just prior to the next inhalation.
Rhythmic breathing	The rider should inhale to a count of 4, hold for a count of 4, exhale to a count of 4, and pause for a count of 4 before repeating.
1:2 ratio	The riders should take a deep breath to a count of 4 and then exhale to a count of 8. If a rider runs out of breath before getting to 8, the next time he or she should take a deeper breath and exhale more slowly. With practice, the counts may need to be altered to 5:10 or 6:12.
5 to 1 count	As the rider takes a deep, slow breath in, they should say the number 5 and then exhale fully. With the next breath in, the rider slowly says the number 4 and "I am more relaxed now than at 5". Repeat until number 1 is reached.
Concentration	The rider should focus attention on the rhythm of breathing. If their mind wanders to something else, focus should be redirected to breathing and letting the thought disappear. With each breath out, the rider should think of becoming more relaxed.

Source: Williams and Harris (2001)

Case Study 2.4

Ann found that she suffered from a lot of stress and anxiety, not only when competing, but also in her everyday life; this was affecting her riding, as she would start stressed, and little things would niggle at her, causing her to overreact.

Her coach suggested a relaxation exercise that she could practice daily (avoiding the first hour after having eaten) to help her generally reduce her levels of stress and anxiety.

- Sit or lie quietly in a comfortable position.
- Close your eyes.
- Starting at your feet and working progressively up to your face, relax all your muscles.
- Breathe through your nose and concentrate on each breath in and out.
- Choose a word that reflects the emotion you would like to be experiencing, such as "calm", or "relaxed", or "chilled", to help keep your attention on your breathing.
- As you breathe out, silently say the word to yourself.
- Continue for 10–20 minutes.
- When you have finished, sit quietly for a few minutes.

Once this has become a familiar routine, an abbreviated version can be used at any time to reduce anxiety. Simply breathe deeply for a few seconds whilst repeating the cue word.

Some disciplines require riders to generate energy and get "psyched up" for competition, and this too is a skill that can be learned and developed. The use of music with a strong beat or physical exercise such as running or jumping on the spot are commonly used methods for increasing energy levels.

Breathing Exercise for Increasing Energy

Start by breathing in a relaxed, regular manner. The rider should imagine with each inhalation they are generating more energy and activation. With each exhalation they are getting rid of any fatigue. The riders can then begin to increase their breathing rate as they increase their level of energy generation. It may help to say "energy in" with each inhalation and "fatigue out" with each exhalation. (Williams and Harris, 2001)

2.4 COGNITIVE CONTROL STRATEGIES

Attention and Concentration Control

Developing verbal or kinaesthetic cues to focus concentration or to re-focus lost concentration also helps to control stress levels. A verbal cue may be a technical instruction to ensure your technique is correct, such as "look up", or simply something to release tension, such as "smile". A kinaesthetic cue may be to re-adjust your riding position or move a part of the body, for example, shrugging shoulders, stretching the legs out of the stirrups, rolling the ankles in order to relax them, or taking a deep breath to release tension.

Most riders will practice riding their dressage test, a show jumping course, or specific fences they might encounter on a cross country course in preparation for a competition. However, many will not practice in the actual clothes or equipment they are likely to be using on the day. For riders (or indeed horses) who are easily distracted, this can provide another opportunity to lose concentration at competitions when the clothes or equipment they are using feel very different. It can also be beneficial to simulate the noise and activity that is likely to be encountered on the show ground (Schmid et al, 2001).

Self Talk

Some of the most common self-defeating attitudes can be categorised as follows:

- Perfectionism: "I must be perfect at all times; I mustn't get this wrong; I mustn't make a mistake."
- Catastrophising: Accompanies perfectionism; a little error becomes a disaster. The rider tends to focus a lot on "what ifs". "What if he stops; What if I forget my test".
- Self-worth tied to achievement: "If I don't win this, I'm useless".
- Personalisation: "A poor mark means I must be a poor rider".
- Blaming: Making excuses or assigning fault to others.
- Black/white thinking: May lead to labeling, for example, "I get really nervous at competitions, therefore I can't cope with pressure".
- Generalisations: Linking a single incident with an inevitable outcome. Going wrong in a dressage test leads to "I told you I can't remember medium tests".

(Gauron, 1984)

The most effective way to combat these negative, debilitating thoughts is to use a method known as "thought stopping", followed by positive self talk and affirmations.

Thought stopping relies on the rider recognising when negative thoughts are entering their mind and using either the word "stop" or imagining a stop sign in their head blocking the path of these thoughts. Other individuals find it easier to use physical movements such as shaking the head or shrugging the shoulders to get rid of negativity. The next step is to insert more positive thoughts and images in their place (Williams and Leffingwell, 1996).

Table 2.13. Changing self talk.

Self-Defeating Thoughts	Positive/Perspective Statement
I can't believe it's raining; the ground is really boggy, and my horse hates the wet.	It's the same for everyone, and I can ride just as well in it – I've had plenty of practice!
I rode like an idiot.	Everyone makes mistakes, and I've just learned how not to do it.
The judging is awful.	It's not in my control. I'll just concentrate on riding the best I can.
I don't want to fall off.	I won't gain anything unless I take risks. I just need to trust my horse and our preparation.
I don't want to let people down.	I can only think about myself and my horse. Providing I do my best and the best for my horse. Then I've done well.
We'll win if I can just jump clear.	Keep focused on riding into each fence as I would at home – forward and balanced.

Zinsser et al (2001) suggest that it may be helpful for riders to make a table with a list of the self-defeating thoughts they commonly use on one side and a positive or perspective-changing statement on the other (Table 2.13).

Imagery

Imagery involves using all the senses to create or recreate an experience in the mind. It is based on the principle that the mind can't tell the difference between what is real and what is imagined. Research indicates that when an individual engages in vivid and absorbing imagery the brain interprets this as identical to the actual event happening.

Simple Exercise for Demonstrating the Power of Imagery

This can be performed mounted or dismounted.

Ask the rider to put their arm out to the side at shoulder height and then take their arm back behind them, twisting at the waist but without moving from the spot. Ask them to go as far as they can and then look down their arm, picking a point such as a tree or fence post to mark how far back their arm went.

Now ask them to return to the starting position, close their eyes, see themselves taking their arm back to the tree or fence post noted, and then going past it to the next tree, fence post, or other marker.

The rider should now open their eyes and repeat the exercise, again aiming to take their arm as far back as possible without moving from the spot. This time the rider will be able to take their arm further back than the first time and will reach the marker they visualised in their mind.

The power of imagery is that it allows riders to practice skills and strategies without physically being on a horse or in the training environment. It can be used by beginners and experienced riders alike to enhance physical, perceptual and psychological skills (Tables 2.14, 2.15 and 2.16).

Guidelines for using imagery effectively are:

- Practice it regularly (five-minute sessions daily are sufficient).
- Use all the senses to improve the vividness of the image and include emotion (i.e., how you are feeling or want to be feeling) into the image.
- Use both internal and external perspectives. For example, see yourself doing the course (as if on video) and then see it through your own eyes riding the course.
- Use imagery in practice and competition.
- Use video/audio tapes to enhance imagery skills.
- Use triggers or cues to facilitate imagery.
- Emphasise dynamic kinaesthetic imagery, that is, the feel of executing the movement.

Table 2.14.   Imagery to enhance physical skills.

Learning sport skills	When used with cue words, imagery can help novice riders to improve their riding technique. Images such as a piece of elastic attached to the top of the riding hat and linked with the words "grow tall" can encourage riders to sit upright.
	Imagining straight lines from the hand to the bit and the hip to the heel are useful tools for ensuring correct positioning of the hands and the legs.
	Imagining holding a bird in the hand, tight enough to prevent escape but relaxed enough that it isn't hurt, gives riders an idea about how to hold the reins.
Practicing sport skills	Imagery can be used to practice a specific skill repetitively in the mind. Dressage riders might use imagery to practice half halts and "seeing" the horse lower its hindquarters.
	Cross country riders might use the image of riding down a tunnel to practice jumping narrow or combination fences.
	Show jumpers might imagine the feeling of a coiled spring that will propel them over the puissance wall.
	In fact, most riders will use imagery during their mental rehearsal to practice their dressage test, show jumping course, or route on the cross country.
Solving technique problems	When riders are experiencing problems with their technique, it can be useful to watch a video of a time when they rode well and internalise the feelings they had during that time. They can then use this to compare to how they currently feel when performing the movement or tackling the fence and note any differences.

Source: Vealey and Greenleaf (2001)

Table 2.15. Imagery to enhance perceptual skills.

Practicing strategy	If a rider knows his horse tends to jump to the left over drop fences or back off going into the water, he can use imagery to rehearse how he is going to deal with it so that if it does happen on competition day, his body can react on autopilot to correct it.
Perceptual problem solving	If a strategy is not working or riders are experiencing problems in their riding, it can be useful to use imagery to think through various options and predict how the horse might react to each and which is most likely to be the solution. Often by relaxing the mind and imagining the situation, the rider can gain a clearer insight and successfully determine how to correct the problem.

Source: Vealey and Greenleaf (2001)

Table 2.16. Imagery to enhance psychological skills.

Arousal control	By recalling the preparation put in before the competition and previous good performances, riders can increase their confidence and reduce their anxiety levels.
Stress management	Riders can aim to have two or three restful and relaxing images they can call on when they start to feel stressed or under pressure. These might be images of a peaceful hack in the country, lying on a beach in the sun, or relaxing in a favourite place. Equally, focusing on symbolic images, such as a twisted rope uncoiling or a block of ice melting, can help to reduce stress.
Increasing self-awareness	By imaging the training sessions or past competitions, riders can become aware of what actually happened and the things they were doing or not doing that directly affected their performance.
Self-confidence	If something hasn't gone well or the rider feels he or she could have ridden better, then imagery can be used to "put it right". The rider should run through a positive version of the round or test by correcting the mistake or successfully negotiating the jump. The rider should think of it as recording over the poor performance in their mind and replacing it with a successful performance.

Source: Vealey and Greeleaf (2001)

- Imagine in real time (avoid speeding up or slowing down the images)
- Keep a log of useful imagery routines and words

(Gould and Damarjian, 1996)

The main obstacles to successful imagery training are the unrealistic expectations of either the coach or the rider, a lack of commitment to practice and a lack of coach follow-up and support.

Case Study 2.5

Dan is a dressage rider who is frustrated because he never seems to ride as well in competition as he does in training. After discussions with his coach and after experimenting with different techniques, he has developed an imagery strategy that enables him to get the most from himself and his horse at competitions.

Firstly, at home he practices the movements individually and pays particular attention to how he and the horse feel. Then after riding, he spends 5–10 minutes daily just going through each movement in his head. He feels how he is riding; what he is doing with his hands, legs, and seat; and what he can see and hear.

As the competition draws near, Dan uses his daily imagery to put the movements together and ride the test from start to finish. He imagines executing all the transitions perfectly and exactly at the marker. He can see the relaxed ears of his horse and hear the lightness and rhythm of the steps. He rides the test through in his mind to the salute at the end and then imagines the feelings of satisfaction as he pats his horse and leaves the arena.

On competition day, he again goes through the test in his head before getting on and warming up. Just before entering the arena he uses the words "aloof expression" to put himself in the right frame of mind to go in and ride calmly, confidently, and with authority.

SUMMARY

- Being able to recognise and manage a rider's emotional and psychological state is an important skill for all coaches.
- The motivation of an individual can be influenced in four key areas: self-efficacy, attributions, orientation and achievement motivation.
- Coaches should provide opportunities for riders to feel successful as well as use strategies such as modelling and positive self talk to enhance self-efficacy.
- Individuals can attribute their success or failure to internally controlled factors such as effort or skill or to externally controlled factors such as task difficulty or luck.
- Coaches should aim to increase feelings of control and competence through the use of internal attributions to explain performance.
- Intrinsically motivated riders are more likely to persist for longer and have greater resilience in times of difficulty.
- Success should not be seen in terms of outcome and winning, but in terms of delivering personal performance.
- A rider can have a long-term aim, supported by long-term, intermediate-, and short-term goals.
- Outcome goals are important for competitions but should always be backed up by performance and process goals which are within the control of the rider.

- Performance profiling is a useful technique for identifying process goals for training and competition.
- The ability of the rider to alter their focus of concentration from broad to narrow and internal to external can have a profound effect on performance.
- Stress and anxiety can manifest in physical, psychological and behavioural symptoms. These can positively or negatively affect performance, depending on whether the rider views them as facilitating or debilitating to their performance.
- Stress and anxiety can be managed through thorough preparation, relaxation exercises, and increased self- efficacy.
- Other cognitive control strategies include the use of verbal and kinaesthetic cues, controlling self talk and imagery.

Self Study

1. Practice at least one relaxation exercise and one cognitive control exercise for 10–15 minutes each day for a week.
2. Undertake a performance profiling exercise with either yourself or a rider that you coach (Appendix 2).

Exam Style Questions

1. Discuss the following statement:
   "Setting the toughest and most challenging goals is the best way to improve performance."
2. Explain the different theories on the effect of arousal on performance and their relevance for the equine coach.
3. Describe three strategies for combating competitive anxiety.
4. Identify four ways in which a coach can influence a rider's motivation. Provide examples of each.

References

Bandura, A. (1997). *Self-efficacy. The exercise of control*. New York: Macmillan.

Boutcher, S.H. and Rotella, R.J. (1987). A psychological skills educational program for closed-skill performance enhancement. *The Sport Psychologist*, 1, 127–137.

Butler, R.J. and Hardy, L. (1992). The performance profile: theory and application. *The Sport Psychologist*, 6, 253–264.

Carver, C.S. and Scheier, M.F. (1988). A control perspective on anxiety. *Anxiety Research*, 1, 17–22.

Dale, G.A. and Wrisberg, C.A. (1996). The use of a performance profiling technique in a team setting: Getting the athletes and coach on the "same page". *The Sport Psychologist*, 10, 261–271.

Davis, B., Roscoe, J., Roscoe, D. and Bull, R. (2005). *Physical Education and the Study of Sport*. Edinburgh: Elsevier Mosby.

Duda, J.L. (1989). Relationship between task and ego orientation and the perceived purpose of sport among high school athletes. *Journal of Sport and Exercise Psychology*, 11, 319–334.

Duda, J.L. and Treasure, D.C. (2001). Toward optimal motivation in sport: Fostering athletes' competence and sense of control. In *Applied Sport Psychology: Personal Growth to Peak Performance* (edited by J.M. Williams), 43–62. California: Mayfield.

Gauron, E.F. (1984). *Mental Training for Peak Performance*. New York: Sport Science Associates.

Gill, D.L. (2000). *Psychological Dynamics of Sport and Exercise*. Champaign, IL: Human Kinetics.

Gould, D. (2001). Goal setting for peak performance. In *Applied Sport Psychology: Personal Growth to Peak Performance* (edited by J.M. Williams), 190–205. California: Mayfield.

Gould, D. and Damarjian (1996). Imagery training for peak performance. In *Exploring Sport and Exercise Psychology* (edited by J.L. Van Raalte and B.W. Brewer), 25–50. Washington: American Psychological Association.

Gould, D., Petlichkoff, L., Hodge, K. and Simons, J. (1990). Evaluating the Effectiveness of a Psychological Skills Educational Workshop. *The Sport Psychologist*, 4, 249–260.

Gould, D. and Weinberg, R. (1995) *Foundations of Sport and Exercise Psychology*. California: Human Kinetics.

Hardy, L. (1996). A test of catastrophe models of anxiety and sports performance against multidimensional anxiety theory models using the method of dynamic differences. *Anxiety, Stress and Coping: An International Journal*, 9, 69–86.

Hardy, L., Jones, G. and Gould, D. (1996). *Understanding Psychological Preparation for Sport: Theory and Practice of Elite Performers*. Chichester, UK: Wiley.

Jones, G. and Swain, A. (1995). Predisposition to experience debilitative and facilitative anxiety in elite and non elite performers. *The Sport Psychologist*, 9, 201–211.

Locke, E.A. and Latham, G.P. (1985). The application of goal setting to sports. *Journal of Sport Psychology*, 7, 205–222.

Martens, R. (1987). *Coaches Guide to Sport Psychology*. Champaign, IL: Human Kinetics.

Martens, R., Vealey, R. and Burton, D. (1990). *Competitive Anxiety*. Champaign, IL: Human Kinetics.

Meyers, M.C., Bourgeois, A.E., LeUnes, A. and Murray, N.G. (1999). Mood and psychological skills of elite and sub-elite equestrian athletes. *Journal of Sport Behaviour*, 22(3), 399–409.

Nideffer, R.M. and Sagal, M.S. (2001). Concentration and attention control training. In *Applied Sport Psychology: Personal Growth to Peak Performance* (edited by J.M. Williams), 312–332. California: Mayfield.

Pierce, B.E. and Burton, D. (1998). Scoring the perfect 10: Investigating the impact of goal-setting styles on a goal setting program for female gymnasts. *Journal of Sport Psychology*, 12, 156–168.

Rotella, R. (1983). Riding out of your mind. *Practical Horseman*, 11(8), 29–31.

Schmid, A., Peper, E. and Wilson, V.E. (2001). Strategies for training concentration. In *Applied Sport Psychology: Personal Growth to Peak Performance* (edited by J.M. Williams), 333–346. California: Mayfield.

Steinberg Horn, T., Lox, C.L. and Labrador, F. (2001). The self-fulfilling prophecy theory: When coaches' expectations become reality. In *Applied Sport Psychology: Personal Growth to Peak Performance* (edited by J.M. Williams), 63–81. California: Mayfield.

Vealey, R.S. and Greenleaf, C.A. (2001). Seeing is believing: understanding and using imagery in sport. In *Applied Sport Psychology: Personal Growth to Peak Performance* (edited by J.M. Williams), 247–272. California: Mayfield.

Weinberg, R.S. and Williams, J.M. (2001). Integrating and implementing a psychological skills training programme. In *Applied Sport Psychology: Personal Growth to Peak Performance* (edited by J.M. Williams), 347–377.

Weiner, B. (1986). *An Attributional Theory of Motivation and Emotion.* New York: Springer-Verlag.

Williams, J.M. and Harris, D.V. (2001). Relaxation and energizing techniques for regulation of arousal. In *Applied Sport Psychology: Personal Growth to Peak Performance* (edited by J.M. Williams), 229–246. California: Mayfield.

Williams, J.M. and Leffingwell, T.R. (1996). Cognitive strategies in sport and exercise psychology. In *Exploring sport and exercise psychology* (edited by J. L.Van Raalte and B.W. Brewer), 51–73. Washington: American Psychological Association.

Zinsser, N., Bunker, L. and Williams, J.M. (2001). Cognitive Techniques for Building Confidence and Enhancing Performance. In *Applied Sport Psychology: Personal Growth to Peak Performance* (edited by J.M. Williams), pp. 284–311. California: Mayfield.

Preparing Effective Coaching Sessions

Chapter Objective

To provide an insight into learning styles, skill acquisition, and the principles of training.

3.1   LEARNING STYLES

A learning style refers to the way an individual perceives, processes, and understands information. Most riders will have a preferred learning style, for example, the rider who likes to hear the coach explain what to do in detail before having a go; the rider who prefers to watch a demonstration of the task before attempting it; or the rider who just wants to have a go and then discuss the exercise later. The difficulty for coaches is that these three riders with their three different learning styles could be taking part in the same coaching session.

Each coach will also have a preferred coaching style, which is strongly influenced by their learning style. In other words, they will tend to coach in the same style as that in which they like to learn. For example, an individual who, when learning new things, prefers to just have a go at an exercise before thinking too much about it, is likely to ask the riders they coach to do the same: "Just jump through this grid and then we'll have a chat about it." This can seriously unsettle those riders who prefer to have a detailed explanation of each exercise before they tackle it. Therefore it is important to be aware of your own preferred style as well as the styles of those you are coaching.

Coaching individuals is a less daunting proposition since the coach can take the time to identify the rider's preferred learning style and then adapt their own style to accommodate it. The ability to do this can help explain why some riders feel they "just click" with their current coach and some feel they are simply not on the same wavelength. The most effective coaching strategy for groups is variability. A coach must be able to use a variety of styles to enable each individual to get as much from the session as possible.

Honey and Mumford (1992) identified four different learning styles; activists, reflectors, theorists and pragmatists (Table 3.1). As the name suggests, activists learn by doing. Their preference is to have a go at new exercises rather than think about them, and they tend to act first and consider the consequences afterwards.

In contrast, reflectors learn through observation. They are cautious and thought-ful individuals who like to consider all the angles and possible outcomes before attempting anything new. Theorists like to understand the theory behind the exercises. They need to know why the exercise is being used, how best to perform it, and what the outcome should be before having a go. Ideally, they would like to see the exercise being executed correctly, either through a demonstration, photos, or video, before putting it into practice themselves.

Pragmatists are keen to try different exercises and tend to look for new strategies or new approaches to problems. They are practical and down-to-earth people who welcome brief instructions but become bored and impatient with long, convoluted discussions. The key to successful coaching of pragmatists is to demonstrate the value in a particular exercise because they dislike doing things just for the sake of doing them.

Each learning style requires a different coaching approach to optimise the learning experience (Table 3.2). Children are a classic example of activists. They generally prefer to work with others, so group coaching is likely to be effective. Learning can be optimised through the use of safe and fun experimentation with new exercises and experiences and challenges or problems to work through. Good examples are

Table 3.1.   Learning styles.

Activists	Learn by doing. Activists like to involve themselves in new experiences and tend to act first and consider the consequences afterwards.
Reflectors	Learn by observation. Reflectors like to consider all the angles and implications and tend to be cautious and thoughtful.
Theorists	Need to understand the theory. Theorists like to understand the theory behind actions. They need facts, figures, models, and concepts and feel uncomfortable with subjective judgements.
Pragmatists	Keen to try things out. Pragmatists look for new ideas and tend to be impatient with long, open-ended discussions. They are practical and down to earth.

Table 3.2. Coaching strategies.

	Learn best when:	**Learn least when:**
Activists	Involved in new experiences Thrown in at the deep end Working with others Problem solving Role playing Taking the lead	Listening to long explanations Reading and thinking on their own Following precise instructions
Reflectors	Able to stand back and observe Given time to think Given opportunity to review Not under pressure	Forced to take the lead Doing things without preparation Rushed
Theorists	Activity is backed up by theory There's a clear structure and purpose Able to question and explore ideas	Emphasis on emotions and feelings There's a lack of structure and purpose Asked to act without understanding principles or concepts
Pragmatist	Shown practical advantages Try things and get feedback Can copy an example or role model	No immediate practical benefit No clear guidelines Appears to be all theory

the use of quadrilles. The group is divided into two and asked to perform exercises where they must pass in opposite directions and come together to ride as pairs down the centre line or change the rein across opposite diagonals between the horses of the other group. These types of exercise promote spatial awareness, control, and co-ordination.

Groups that include activists and reflectors work well because the activists can get on and try the exercises while the reflectors observe. Reflectors function well when they are allowed to absorb the information being given and have time to process and review this information before attempting the exercise. The worst type of situation for reflectors is one where they feel under pressure, rushed, or forced to take the lead.

Theorists tend to, typically, represent the learning style of the majority of adult riders. They like to have the theory behind the exercises explained and the opportunity to discuss and explore ideas as well as to ask questions. These individuals function best when there is a clear structure and purpose to the coaching session.

Pragmatists need to be shown why a particular exercise is useful and how it will benefit them and their horses. They like to have clear guidelines about how to execute the exercise and, ideally, an opportunity to see an example of correct execution. They then want the opportunity to have a go and get feedback.

Case Study 3.1 demonstrates how a coach can organise their coaching sessions to accommodate the different learning styles exhibited by each member of the group.

Case Study 3.1

Kate is taking a cross country training session with four riders of the local riding club event team. She has coached them before and knows that Ben likes challenges and just wants to have a go *(activist)*; John prefers to watch the others take their turn and then have a go himself *(reflector)*; Tony wants a brief explanation about what he is aiming for and the opportunity to ask questions before attempting the exercise *(theorist)*; and Jill likes one or two key points to focus on that will enable her to ride the exercise successfully *(pragmatist)*.

At the water jump she asks Ben to go through first and then uses his example as an opportunity to review what went well and what could be done differently, and then to add a few key points on how to ride water jumps. She then asks if there are any questions and suggests that Tony go next, followed by Jill, and lastly John.

Kolb's Learning Cycle

Kolb (1984) identified four learning styles and incorporated them into a learning cycle as shown in Figure 3.1. This model suggests that to learn effectively an individual needs to move around the cycle. The learning begins with the individual experiencing an exercise. Next, the individual must think about and review the exercise and draw conclusions about what happened during it. Finally, they must decide what to do in the future execution of the exercise. The rider then returns to the beginning of the cycle, and the process starts again. Completing each stage is important because it improves the quality of the learning in the next stage.

This cycle is true for both those learning or improving their riding skills as well as coaches aiming to improve their coaching skills. The first step is always to participate in or deliver an exercise. The second step is to review what happened

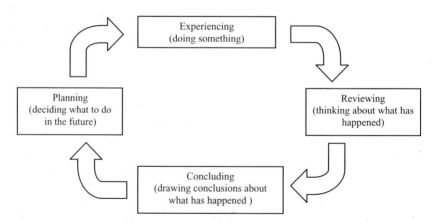

Figure 3.1   Learning cycle.

during the execution of the exercise: what went well, what didn't go well, and if it achieved the desired outcome. Conclusions are then drawn, and a decision is made on the next step in the coaching process. This might be deciding how to modify the exercise, identifying the next progressive exercise, or deciding to try something completely different. This process can happen in the space of a one-hour coaching session or may take several days to complete, depending on the experience, awareness, and ability of the coach.

Interestingly, this cycle can easily be related to Honey and Mumford's model.

Experiencing = Activist
Reviewing = Reflector
Concluding = Theorist
Planning = Pragmatist

A coach who has a preference for an activist style of learning may provide plenty of new experiences for their riders but fail to reflect on, draw conclusions from, and build on these experiences. A coach whose style is predominantly a reflector may be good at reviewing what is happening during an exercise but may find it difficult to draw conclusions and make decisions about what to do next. They are likely to function well when everything is going to plan, but may struggle to instantly come up with solutions when things go wrong.

Those who demonstrate a theorist style are likely to have lots of ideas about how and why things happen during the exercise but may spend more time discussing and theorising than actually providing opportunities to practice exercises. The pragmatist coach is likely to avoid theoretical discussion and instead concentrate on reviewing why a particular exercise is useful. These coaches can lose patience with riders who may want to know exactly how and why an exercise works. They like the results to speak for themselves.

When coaches are aware of their preferred and least preferred styles, they can identify their strengths and weaknesses within the learning cycle and adapt their coaching sessions accordingly.

The models outlined above demonstrate that throughout the learning process different approaches are required in order for learning to be effective. Therefore, it is important for riders and coaches to be as flexible as possible and to develop their skills in using other styles to maximise their own learning and that of others.

Informational Styles

Before coaches can start their riders on the "experiencing" stage of the learning cycle, they must provide riders with information and instructions about what to do. Again, each individual will have a preferred method of receiving information, and this will affect their ability to understand and act upon the information. Equally, it will also affect the coach's delivery of the information as they will tend to give information in their preferred style of receiving it. These informational styles fall into four categories: auditory, visual, kinaesthetic, and thinking (Table 3.3). There are some obvious similarities with the four learning styles previously identified.

Table 3.3. Informational styles.

Auditory learners	Learn best through hearing. They benefit from spoken instructions, talking things out, and the use of keywords.
Visual learners	Learn best through seeing. They benefit from visual aids, demonstrations, and written explanations.
Kinaesthetic learners	Learn through doing. They benefit from "hands on" activities and process information through movement, body language, and gestures.
Thinking learners	Learn through analysing movement, principles, skills, and strategies. They like to solve movement problems by asking questions and use their creativity to come up with solutions.

In order to identify an individual's informational style, the coach can look for various clues in the way they act and talk. Table 3.4 lists some of the characteristics of each style and suggests the type of language used for each. The coach can incorporate these words and phrases into the way they give out information and instructions and as a result increase the understanding and rapport between themselves and their riders.

In addition, there are a number of coaching strategies that will appeal to each informational style (Table 3.5). Individuals whose preference is to receive information visually like to see exercises being performed either by demonstration, photographs, or videos. They also find written information useful. For these riders the coach can suggest background reading, attending lecture demonstrations, watching appropriate videos or DVDs or can provide written notes on the coaching sessions.

Visual perception is considered to be the most important source of information when performing sports skills. However, the coach should not assume that the rider knows what to look for. Therefore they should provide clear indicators about what to look for and what constitutes good and poor performance.

Those with a preference for an auditory informational style like to talk about the exercises and get verbal feedback on how they are doing. Coaches should provide ample opportunity for discussion during their sessions, encourage the riders to summarise instructions, and suggest they make time to discuss the exercises with other riders after the session. Auditory riders also tend to focus on sounds and rhythms to learn movement patterns. In this situation coaches should emphasis the sound of the footfalls, flapping of the mane in a relaxed, even rhythm, and the breathing rhythm of the horse and rider.

The individual who prefers to receive information kinaesthetically needs plenty of opportunity to practice and experiment. Whilst verbal instruction from the coach is essential, it should be short and concise with the use of key action words to focus the rider's attention on the feel of the exercise. Information is actually processed by these riders when they are given the opportunity to move. The coach needs to provide opportunities to practice movements in a structured manner, giving clear direction about the correct execution of the exercises. Simulating actual competition activities are highly effective.

Table 3.4. Informational style characteristics.

	Characteristics	**Useful phrases**
Visual learners	Well organised Observant Neat, well groomed, and orderly Appearance is important Fast talkers Use quick, expressive gestures	Let's have a look at. . . . Show me. . . . Watch out for. . . . Focus on. . . . Imagine you are. . . . Observe the way. . . . Visualise. . . . Appear to be. . . .
Auditory learners	Tend to talk to themselves Easily distracted by noise Very talkative Love discussions May monopolise conversations Usually like music and talking on the phone Tend to carry head to one side	Listen to the rhythm. Let's talk it through. Remark on the. . . . Describe in detail. . . . Hear the. . . . Comment on. . . . Tune in to. . . . Tell me about. . . .
Kinaesthetic learners	Often move and talk slowly Use action words Tend to stand closer to people Use a lot of controlled gestures Move frequently Tend to fidget Often look down Generally have a relaxed posture	Feel the. . . . Give the impression of. . . . Experience the feeling. . . . Demonstrate how to. . . . Practice using the. . . . Try to. . . . How do you feel. . . .

Thinking learners	Talkative
	Like to band ideas about
	Fast moving, thinking and
	   talking
	Like to ask lots of questions
	Come up with creative and
	   innovative ideas for solving
	   problem
		Analyse the differences in. . . .
		Examine why. . . .
		Investigate how. . . .
		Compare the movement. . . .
		Explore how. . . .

The rider who prefers a thinking style requires information that they can analyse to enable them to understand the principles behind the movement. They can be considered the academics of the riding world. Coaches need to provide opportunities for these riders to process information in a variety of ways, including providing scientific articles to read, in-depth discussion, and analysing the movement of horses and riders and the outcomes of competitions. The use of challenging questions of "why" and "how" before and after practice can prove hugely stimulating for these individuals.

Table 3.5. Coaching strategies.

Visual	Auditory	Kinaesthetic	Thinking
Provide visual feedback, such as photos, videos, and demonstrations of what happened. Arrange situations where learners can see things in order to better understand them. Provide opportunities to watch others. Suggest background reading, attending a lecture or demonstration, or provide videos to watch.	Provide regular feedback, as these learners like to be told how they're doing. Provide ample opportunity for discussion. Use verbal instructions. Encourage individuals to repeat and summarise instructions. Encourage individuals to talk to other riders.	Use action words. Talk in a controlled and considered manner. Allow plenty of time to practise. Provide opportunities to experiment.	Provide opportunities to analyse the movement. Encourage individuals to find solutions to riding problems. Allow plenty of time for questions. Provide information individuals can evaluate.

It is suggested that the general population is made up of 45% visual learners, 10% auditory learners, 40% kinaesthetic learners, and 5% thinking learners. This suggests that as coaches we should be limiting what is said (auditory) to the essential instructions and key words and maximising what is seen (visual) and experienced (kinaesthetic).

Case Study 3.2

Lee is running a session for a group of students on riding counter canter.

Firstly, he gives brief instructions about the exercise they will be doing.

"Pick up canter on the right rein, and at M ride across the diagonal, returning to the track between E and K. Counter canter for a few strides, then do a transition to trot before the corner". *(Auditory)*

He then walks the exercise out on the arena to show the riders where they should be riding the movement and where to aim. *(Visual)*. He uses this opportunity to verbally summarise the information he has just given.

"OK, have a go and let me know how it feels." *(Kinaesthetic)*

After each rider has completed the exercise *(experiencing)*, Lee asks them to reflect on what went well and what they would do differently next time *(reviewing)*.

Once everybody has attempted the exercise, Lee summarises the general points that came out of the reviews *(concluding)* and then gives each individual something specific to work on for their second go at the exercise *(planning)*.

Table 3.6.   Barriers to learning.

Psychological factors	Anxiety, lack of motivation, boredom, negative self talk can be barriers to learning.
Physical fitness	Fatigue, lack of appropriate fitness, lack of physical ability can limit learning.
Changes in technique	As riders focus on a new tactic or aspect of technique, they may experience a temporary deterioration in their performance. This can be unsettling, especially if every time they learn something new, they find their performance (albeit temporarily) dropping. As a result the rider may be reluctant to learn new things.
Changes in cognitive strategy	The way in which a rider thinks about a skill can affect learning. If this is changed, such as by introducing a new visualisation technique, performance can be affected. Until this new cognitive strategy reaches the autonomous stage, the rider may well see deterioration in performance and may prove reluctant in the future to try new strategies.
Personal life	Changes in a rider's personal life can affect the ability and motivation to learn. Relationship, money, and work or school worries can all have an impact.

Source: Christina and Corcos (1988)

Case Study 3.2 effectively demonstrates how both the learning cycle and an appreciation of riders' informational styles can be incorporated into the coaching session to optimise learning for all involved. However, despite the best efforts of the coach to provide an environment that caters to all learning and informational styles, there may be other factors that limit or prevent the rider from learning (Table 3.6). Psychological and physical factors, as well as changes in technique, cognitive strategy, and in a rider's personal life, can all impact on their ability to learn.

3.2   EQUINE LEARNING

It is pertinent at this point to highlight a few areas of equine learning that a coach should be aware of. Horses are constantly modifying their behaviour as a result of experience, and the impact of these experiences should be judged not by the motive of the rider (or coach), but by the reaction of the horse. How a horse perceives an action will determine how it reacts in the future (Mills, 1998).

When learning a new exercise, it is likely that the horse will make mistakes. If these mistakes are viewed as annoying and unacceptable by the rider or coach, they may punish the horse, causing anxiety and confusion. However, if these incorrect responses are ignored and only the correct response rewarded, the mistakes eventually decrease in frequency. Simultaneously, the correct response, because it has been rewarded, will increase in frequency and replace the incorrect responses (McCall, 1990).

Research has shown that horses learn best if training sessions are kept short. Long training sessions lead to inefficient learning. Ideally, the horse should work on a different skill each day, and once they have performed the skill successfully a couple of times, it should move on to the next task. Whilst this does increase the time taken to achieve a particular level of performance, the actual performance is of a higher quality (Rubin et al, 1980; McCall et al, 1993).

It is equally important to keep horses learning new tasks rather than just practicing the established ones. This is because horses "learn to learn". The more tasks a horse learns to perform (whether they are relevant for competition or not), the easier it is for the horse to learn subsequent new tasks (McCall, 1990).

As many riders and coaches will be aware, horses have difficulty replacing previous learning with new learning, so any bad habits that have developed are hard to eradicate. However, this is equally true of good habits, and thus a strong emphasis on the correct basic training and positive training experiences in the early stages is essential – first learned is best learned (Sappington et al, 1997).

The implications of this research for the coach is that what is best for the rider in terms of their training may not be what is best for the horse. There are two athletes to consider. A rider just learning to ride a half pass is best partnered with an experienced dressage horse who is established in the movement and thus less likely to be affected by the inevitable mistakes the rider will make during the learning process. Equally, a horse who is itself just learning to half pass is best partnered with an experienced rider who knows what to reward and what to ignore.

3.3 SKILL ACQUISITION

A skill is the ability to do something; that is, it is something that a person possesses. In sport, skill is considered in three areas: cognitive, perceptual, and motor (Table 3.7). Cognitive skills reflect the ability to think about and solve problems intellectually. Perceptual skills relate to the ability to sense and interpret what is happening and why. Motor skills are those involved in the movement of the body. Sports psychology deals with developing cognitive skills through psychological skills training. Perceptual and motor skills are generally lumped together and referred to as *psychomotor skills*, the ability to sense and interpret information and then to act through movement.

The acquisition of the psychomotor skills necessary to be able to ride follows three phases: the thinking or cognitive stage, the practice or associative stage, and the automatic or autonomous stage (Table 3.8). These are not three distinct phases

Table 3.7. Sport skill.

Cognitive skill	Ability to solve problems by thinking
Perceptual skill	Process by which things are sensed and interpreted
Motor skill	Voluntary movement

Table 3.8.   Phases of psychomotor learning.

Cognitive phase	Rider has to figure out what to do. Trial and error is interspersed with feedback. Conscious attention is paid to detail.	Verbal explanations and demonstrations are important. Problem solving can be useful: "Why do you think I put my weight back like that?"
Associative phase	The rider understands what is required and is now able to start refining skills. The rider is using visual checks less and developing a "feel" for the movement.	Feedback should be specific and focus on what the rider did and what the result was. This allows the association of kinaesthetic feedback with outcomes.
Autonomous phase	Action has become automatic. Rider can now concentrate on the external demands of the environment.	There is less feedback from the coach. Often the coach's role is more facilitative at this stage. This is the stage when riders are likely to be competing successfully.

Source: Fischman and Oxendine (2001)

where a rider moves from one to another, but a description of the process of skill acquisition.

During the cognitive phase, the riders are thinking about what they need to do and attempting to gain an understanding about how to do it. The coach must provide a description and explanation of how the task is to be performed. They may also provide diagrams, videos, or demonstrations to allow the rider to form a visual picture of the skill they are trying to acquire. The riders in this stage will often talk themselves through the exercises using key words and phrases as a reminder of the important points in the process, for example, "sit up, look up, wait for the fence".

Because this early stage in learning requires the full concentration of the rider, they are unable to pay attention to other aspects of the environment such as what the horse is looking at or what other riders are doing. The coach must be aware of this and refrain from admonishing riders for not looking where they are going or for not being prepared when the horse spooks. It is likely the coach will have much better awareness about what is going on around them than the riders, and a few well-placed reminders such as, "look out for Sophie on your left", or "keep your leg on Murphy in the top corner", can pre-empt any incidents. Depending on the skill level of the rider, the cognitive stage may be relatively short. Once the task can be executed to the coach's satisfaction, the rider can now begin practising it.

The associative stage is a much longer phase involving practising the skill until it can be performed accurately and consistently. At this time, the coach's role is to provide suitable practice opportunities for the riders to develop the skill. The rider's attention is taken up less and less by the physical execution of the skill. As

Table 3.9. Practical application of skill acquisition.

Instructing	The "telling phase" gives enough information to allow riders to understand the task.
	Explain what the riders are learning as well as how to execute the task.
	Instruct verbally, but if appropriate, suggest reading theory or use diagrams or videos.
	Present the information clearly and concisely to avoid information overload.
	Use key words for the riders to focus on.
	Start simple. Refinement can be added later.
	Link learning to skills the rider already possesses; for example, ride the show jumps as you would a skinny combination on the cross country.
Demonstrating	Make sure that the rider understands what the exercise should look like and what the purpose of the exercise is.
	Supply the rider with a "model" to aim for.
Applying	Provide the opportunity for the rider to practise the skill.
	Allow plenty of time for this phase.
	Structure the practise effectively so that riders learn to apply what they have learned from instruction and demonstration.
Confirming	This is the process of reviewing and feedback.
	An important aspect of this is to question the rider about what has been learned and what progress has been made.
	This reinforces the learning, helps the coach to confirm the learning objectives have been met, and also encourages the rider to self-evaluate.

Source: Davis et al (2005)

it becomes more automated, the rider can begin to broaden their attention to other aspects of the environment. This might include making better use of the arena, planning where and when to ride the exercises, responding to feedback from the horse, working around other riders, and increasing awareness of outside distractions that could impact on the successful completion of the exercise.

The autonomous phase is the advanced stage of learning. This is the stage at which the rider is able to perform the skill automatically. In fact, if the coach were to ask riders to consciously focus on their movements, it would likely seriously disrupt their performance. The rider is now able to attend fully to what is going on around them and act on the feedback they receive from the horse and the environment. At this stage it is the coach's role to help the riders maintain their level of skill and to motivate them to want to continue to learn and improve.

The practical application of the phases of skill acquisition is detailed in Table 3.9. The cognitive phase requires the coach to instruct and demonstrate the skill. The associative stage requires the coach to provide opportunities for the rider to apply what they have learnt and confirm that they have learnt it. The final, autonomous stage requires the coach to continue to apply and confirm the learning of the skill, but it is likely to be to a lesser extent and at the specific request of the rider.

Case Study 3.3

Anne is taking a team training session for a group of talented junior dressage riders. After the warm-up, she asks the group to line up in the centre of the arena so she can explain the aim of the session.

"Today we are going to work on contact. The aim is to be able to maintain an even and consistent contact whatever exercise is being performed. So what can anybody tell me about contact?"

Once the riders have had a chance to throw in their ideas, she asks one of the riders to come forward and halt side on (in profile) to the group. She then summarises the key points that came out of the discussion and demonstrates how the contact between hand and bit should look.

"See the straight line between the elbow, wrist and bit? Your arms should be against your side, shoulders relaxed and down, and the hands forward towards the horse's mouth."

The rider is asked to rejoin the ride, and Anne moves down the line to demonstrate how the contact should feel. With each horse she takes hold of the reins between the rider's hand and the bit. She then asks the rider to pretend their hands are the horse's mouth and her hands are the rider's hands. She demonstrates what the contact with the horse's mouth should feel like. She then asks each of them to pretend they are the horse trying to evade the contact and demonstrates how the contact should follow the horse's movements.

"So remember, think forward with the hands and allow the contact to follow wherever the horse's head goes."

"OK, let's start by riding around the outside of the arena in walk."

The exercise progresses to riding round the arena in trot and canter. Once everybody has had a good chance to practice in all three paces, Anne calls them back into the middle of the arena and asks the following questions.

"So how did that feel? How did if affect the horse's way of going? How did it affect your riding?"

"We are now going to try 20-metre circles, changing the rein across the diagonal and through two half-20-metre circles. First in walk and then trot."

The riders spend 15 minutes doing this exercise and then return to the centre of the arena. Anne again asks the same questions and reiterates certain key points to each rider as appropriate.

"Okay, now we're going to try maintaining the contact through transitions. You can use the outside of the arena, circles, or changes of direction to do transitions between walk, trot, and canter."

When Anne feels they have had sufficient time to practice, she calls them back into the centre to conclude the session.

"So, today we focused on contact and concentrated on keeping the shoulders relaxed and down, the arms by the side, and the hands forward towards the bit. We also concentrated on maintaining an even contact with a following hand."

All the riders in turn are then asked to comment on what they had learned and what they would be taking away with them.

Anne ended the session by thanking the group for their efforts.

The type of practice session demonstrated in Case Study 3.3 is referred to as distributed practice and is widely regarded as being the most effective form of practice. Distributed practice splits the total practice session into several shorter periods with intervals between them. These intervals can be used for review, feedback, or mental rehearsal.

3.4 PRINCIPLES OF TRAINING

Most riders invest a great deal of time and effort getting their horses fit but pay little attention to their own fitness, even though it may directly affect the horse's way of going. At this point it is useful to clarify what is meant by fitness. A rider does not need to be able to run a marathon or climb a mountain, but they do need to be fit to ride. Just as a sprinter may be fit to run the 100 metres but not the 10,000 metres, a rider may be fit to ride novice dressage tests but not to go three-day eventing. Clearly, the type and level of fitness required varies between sports and disciplines. The main principle is that riders should view themselves, as well as their horses, as athletes.

Physical Fitness

Physical fitness is usually categorised into two areas: health-related fitness and skill-related fitness (Figure 3.2). Health-related fitness includes cardiovascular fitness, muscular strength, muscular endurance, flexibility, and body composition (Table 3.10).

Cardiovascular Fitness

Cardiovascular (CV) fitness is the ability of the heart and lungs to deliver oxygen to the working muscles. The muscles require oxygen to break down glucose and

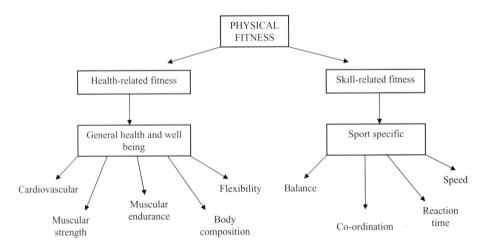

Figure 3.2 Components of physical fitness.

Table 3.10.   Health-related fitness.

Cardiovascular fitness	Also referred to as endurance/aerobic capacity. The ability to exercise the body for long periods of time without fatigue.
Muscular strength	The ability of the muscle to exert a force for a short period of time.
Muscular endurance	The ability to use the muscles repeatedly over a period of time without fatigue.
Flexibility	The range of movement possible at a joint.
Body composition	The percentage of body weight that is lean mass (muscle, bone, vital tissue and organs) and fat mass.

release energy in the form of ATP (adenosine triphosphate). This is called the aerobic energy system and is the most efficient way of producing energy for sustained periods of time.

When training to increase cardiovascular fitness, the aim is to improve the body's ability to get oxygen into the lungs, transfer this oxygen from the lungs into the blood, and then deliver the oxygen via the blood into the working muscles. The more efficient the body is at doing this, the longer it can exercise.

The anaerobic energy system produces ATP from glucose without using oxygen; however, as a result, it also creates a waste by-product called lactic acid. The buildup of lactic acid in the muscles causes a burning sensation and leads to fatigue. The longer the body can keep using the aerobic system to produce energy, the longer it can exercise without the buildup of lactic acid, and therefore without becoming fatigued. In other words, increasing an individual's cardiovascular fitness will increase the amount of time they can exercise before tiring.

Gunning and Graham (1997) highlighted the considerable cardiovascular demands of eventing by demonstrating that event riders on the cross country day of a three-day event maintain high heart rate intensities (up to 90% of their maximum heart rate) for over an hour. Polo players and jockeys are also likely to experience similar heart rate intensities, although probably over a shorter period of time. In contrast, endurance riders, who regularly dismount and run sections of the course, need high levels of cardiovascular fitness and the stamina to maintain this over a prolonged period of time.

Show jumpers and dressage riders are unlikely to require the same levels of aerobic fitness, but they do require light body weight and good muscle tone. Aerobic capacity is likely to be a factor in determining riding performance in competition; therefore, coaches should encourage their riders to undertake some form of physical fitness training in addition to their regular riding (Devienne and Guezennec, 2000; Meyers, 2006).

A simple indicator of cardiovascular fitness is to measure resting heart rate. The resting heart rate will vary depending on the sex, age, health, and fitness of the individual. Those involved in endurance sports will have much lower rates than normal, sometimes as low as 30 beats per minute. This is because their hearts are stronger and able to pump more blood in fewer beats than a less fit person.

Simple Measure of Cardiovascular Fitness: Resting Heart Rate

The best time to measure the resting heart rate is first thing in the morning, just before sitting up to get out of bed.

Find the pulse in the neck or wrist and count the number of beats for 1 minute (or count for 15 seconds and multiply by 4).

The lower the resting heart rate, the better the cardiovascular fitness. An untrained heart would be expected to have a resting rate of about 75 beats per minute (bpm) and a trained heart 60 bpm. (See Appendix 3.)

Riders can improve their cardiovascular fitness by swimming, running, skipping, cycling, or rowing. This type of exercise should be undertaken three to five times per week for 20–60 minutes at a time. Exercise intensity should be moderate so that riders are able to hold a conversation whilst exercising. If an individual is breathing so hard that it is difficult to talk, then he or she is exercising too hard.

Muscular Strength and Muscular Endurance

Muscular strength is the amount of force a muscle can exert against a resistance, for example, lifting a weight or pushing an opponent. This type of strength is less important in riding than it is when doing the various tasks around the stable yard, such as lifting hay or shaving bales. Muscular endurance, however, is an essential part of effective riding. It is important in any activity that requires the same muscle groups to be used repetitively for a prolonged period of time.

In riding it is the abdominal muscles that require high levels of muscular endurance to provide good posture – this is commonly referred to as core stability.

Simple Measure of Abdominal Muscular Endurance: Sit-Ups

Perform as many sit-ups as possible in 30 seconds.

Lie on the floor, with knees bent and arms crossed over the chest (Figure 3.3). Each sit-up begins with the back on the floor. Sit up to the 90-degree position and then return to the floor.

Doing 15–20 sit-ups in 30 seconds is about average.

Riders can improve their core stability through Yoga, Pilates, and exercises using a fitball.

Flexibility

Flexibility, or suppleness, is the range of motion possible at a joint. Individuals can have good flexibility in one area of the body, such as the shoulders, yet have poor

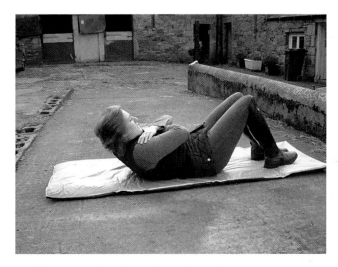

Figure 3.3 Simple measure of abdominal muscular endurance.

flexibility in others, such as the hips or lower limbs. Suppleness is improved by stretching the muscles, tendons, and ligaments beyond their normal range of motion and holding for 10–20 seconds, then resting and repeating.

Riders particularly require flexibility in their hip, knee, and ankle joints. This involves stretching the calf muscles, hamstrings (back of thigh and buttocks), quadriceps (front of thigh), and hip adductors (inner thigh). In addition, most disciplines require a degree of flexibility in the shoulders and lower back.

Simple Measure Of Flexibility: Sit and Reach Test

Sit in front of a step or similar object. Place the feet flat against its surface, keeping the legs straight.

Place a ruler on the top of the step so that it extends 15 cm over the end of the step, with the zero end extending towards you. Reach slowly forward towards the step as far as possible and hold (Figure 3.4).

The coach should read off the distance in centimetres where the outstretched fingertips touch the ruler.

An average score is 7–11 cm.

All riders will benefit from a general flexibility exercise programme such as Yoga or Pilates.

Body Composition

Too little or too much fat on the body can cause problems, particularly for the athlete. A certain amount of fat is necessary as it provides essential fatty acids (a

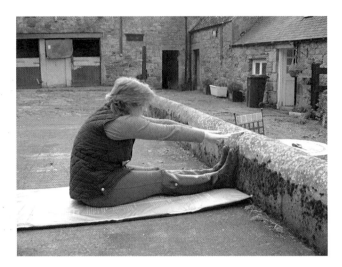

Figure 3.4 Simple measure of flexibility.

rich source of energy) and helps to cushion the internal organs. Too much fat, however, means that the body is carrying unnecessary weight, which can result in extra strain on muscles, joints, and the cardiovascular system. In most sports the higher the percentage of fat, the poorer the performance.

Simple Measure of Body Composition: Body Mass Index

The body mass index (BMI) is a useful measure of body composition.

Record your weight in kilograms and height in metres. Divide the weight by the height squared (BMI = W/H^2).

A healthy BMI range is 19–25.

For most riders it is sufficient to have a BMI within the healthy range. However, jockeys are required to maintain a low body weight and have precise control of their weight during competition. An Australian research study identified that the majority of jockeys found it hard to maintain their riding weight and regularly resorted to extreme and unhealthy practices such as restricting food intake, skipping meals, sauna-induced sweating, and diuretics. These practices should not be condoned as they can lead to severe dehydration, increasing the risk of accident and injury to both horse and jockey (Moore et al, 2002).

Skill-Related Fitness

Skill-related fitness includes balance, co-ordination, reaction time, and speed (Table 3.11). Balance relates to the ability of the rider to maintain equilibrium during move-

Table 3.11.   Skill-related fitness.

Balance	The ability to retain equilibrium (to keep balanced over the centre of gravity) whether stationary or moving.
Co-ordination	The ability to use two or more parts of the body simultaneously.
Reaction time	The time it takes for an individual to respond to a signal.
Speed	The ability to perform a movement quickly, either with the whole body or part of the body.

ment, that is, being able to keep balanced over the centre of gravity on the flat and over fences and through all paces, movements, and changes of direction.

Co-ordination is the ability to use two or more body parts at the same time, such as when using the seat, leg, and reins aids simultaneously to achieve a half halt. Reaction time is the ability of the rider to react quickly to changes in the environment or the horse. This is closely linked to speed, which is the ability of the rider to move quickly with either part or the whole of their body, for instance, being able to get the weight back quickly if the horse pecks on landing after a fence.

All elements of skill-related fitness are sport and discipline specific. It is essential to practice actual activities and movements that will be needed in competition for the rider to truly develop the skill-related fitness required to be successful in their chosen discipline. This means that training to improve skill-related fitness needs to be predominantly carried out on the horse.

Balance

A balanced posture is particularly important for the rider. Balance can be improved by riding on the lunge and riding without stirrups, as well as by using ridden exercises such as grid work and riding over varied terrain. Vaulting is also becoming popular for developing balance in younger riders and should probably be considered as a useful addition to the training programmes of all riders (Figure 3.5).

Simple Measure of Balance: The Stork Stand

Stand straight and evenly on both feet with hands on the hips.

Lift one leg and place the toes against the knee of the other leg (Figure 3.6).

Once secure in this position, raise the heel and stand on the toes for as long as possible without letting the heel touch the floor or the other foot move away from the knee.

Time the balance in seconds.

An average score is between 20 and 30 seconds.

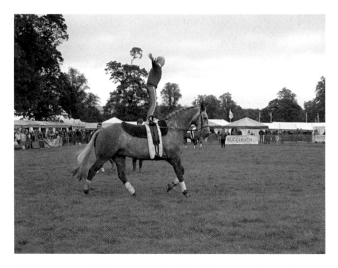

Figure 3.5   Vaulting is a useful exercise to develop balance and co-ordination.

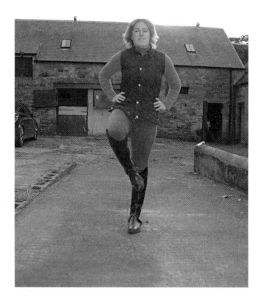

Figure 3.6   Simple measure of balance.

Co-ordination

Co-ordination between a rider's body, seat, leg, and hand is vital for effective communication with the horse. Improving co-ordination can be done by riding and receiving coaching on a school master, riding through grids, riding over varied terrain, and vaulting. Children are generally provided greater opportunities for improving their co-ordination and balance through activities such as Pony Club games and riding quadrilles.

Simple Measure of Co-ordination: Hand Ball Wall Test

Stand 2 m away from a wall.

With the right hand throw a tennis ball against the wall and catch it in the left hand. Then throw with the left hand and catch with the right.

Do this as quickly as possible for 30 seconds.

An average score is 25–30 catches.

Sadly, due to the increasing worry over litigation, the practices of riding without stirrups, riding bareback, and jumping through grids without reins are being used less and less. Providing they are done responsibly and safely, these activities are great opportunities to develop balance, co-ordination, and confidence. In reality, it is unlikely that there will be a resurgence of such exercises, so sports such as vaulting are essential to help develop these skills on the horse.

Reaction Time

The ability to react quickly is important when riding. Whether it is to prevent the horse spooking or to anticipate a stop or run out at a fence, riders need to develop their ability to react quickly and effectively to whatever the horse does.

The best way to develop this ability is to ride as many different horses as possible over varied terrain and in all disciplines. (Computer games can also provide opportunities to improve an individual's reaction time!).

Speed

In the traditional sense of the word – being able to cover a certain distance as quickly as possible – speed has little relevance to the rider. However, when considering polo, eventing, or show jumping, the ability of the rider to move their upper body quickly is a distinct advantage. For example, negotiating a coffin on a cross country course, a jump-off track in a show jumping competition, or rapidly changing direction in a polo match. It may be better to use the term *agility*, which reflects the ability to be able to move the body quickly but in a controlled manner.

The best way to train a rider's ability to move their upper body quickly and effectively is by practising the movements they are likely to need to perform in competition. For the show jumper this may mean grid work and practising the turns and changes of direction required in a jump off. For the event rider this might mean practising jumping drops and combinations, as well as turns and changes of direction. For the polo player this will involve stick and ball exercises during changes of speed and direction. Initially, this can be done at slower speeds but should gradually build up to competition speed.

Fitness Testing

There are a wide range of exercise tests available to quantify both the health- and skill-related fitness of athletes. Many of these methods are often time consuming and require the use of special equipment. A more practical approach is the use of profiling (see Chapter 2). Profiling allows the coach and the rider to identify which elements of fitness are important for their discipline and highlight areas needing improvement in both the horse and the rider. A training programme can then be developed. Case Study 3.4 provides an example of profiling the fitness demands on the rider in calf roping.

Case Study 3.4

Subject: Rodeo athlete
Discipline: Calf roping
Duration of event: 8–10 seconds

The Event

1. Calf is released from chute.
2. Roper gives chase and attempts to throw a rope over the calf's head.
3. Roper dismounts and sprints to the calf.
4. Roper gets control of the calf, lifts and turns it so that it is lying on its back.
5. Roper pulls three of the calf's legs together and ties up.

Demands

Speed: required to dismount and sprint to secure calf after it is roped; required in hands, along with co-ordination to rope and tie the calf.
Muscular strength: required when roping, pinning down, and tying the calf.
Skill work: high demand for skill in roping calf (balance, co-ordination, agility) (see Appendix 3).

(Raether et al, 2000)

Both the coach and rider should both be involved in profiling the demands of the discipline and then using this profile to judge against the rider's current levels of fitness. Although not wholly scientific, it does provide a good base for starting to develop a rider-specific and a discipline-specific fitness training programme.

Types of Training

There are many different types of training that can be used to improve the fitness of both horse and rider.

Continuous Training

Continuous training involves working at the same pace for between 30 minutes and two hours. This activity is usually of moderate intensity and helps improve stamina, health-related fitness, and reduce body fat. For riders this might include running, swimming, or cycling. For horses this is the traditional method of long, slow distance work used in basic fittening.

Cross-Training

Cross-training involves using sports or activities other than the horse and rider's main discipline to improve fitness. Riders who swim, run, or cycle to get fit to ride are cross-training. Dressage horses undertaking grid work, hacking, or cross country are also using cross-training to provide variety and prevent overuse injuries.

Interval Training

Interval training is a common term used in the training of horses today. It consists of alternating periods of hard work with rest periods. These rest periods are essential to allow the body to recover. The aim of interval training is to improve anaerobic and aerobic fitness by varying the work interval's time, distance, intensity, or number of repetitions. It is generally reserved for the specialist training of competition horses. Trainers of racehorses and top level event horses will intersperse periods of fast canter and gallop work with a walk and rest period. The walk period allows the horse's heart rate to return to 110 beats per minute or below before another work period is commenced. Clearly, for this type of training a heart rate monitor should be used.

   Other types of interval training include gridwork, where jumping down the grid is the work period, or hillwork, where cantering up the hill is the work period and walking back down the hill is the rest period.

Fartlek Training

Fartlek training is a system known as "speed play". It involves varying the speed and intensity of the work and terrain covered. With human athletes it relies on the individuals making decisions about how they feel and therefore how fast or slow they will go. The coach can use this method to prevent boredom in the work by encouraging horses and riders to hack out over different types of terrain and allow the horse and rider to choose their own comfortable speed (within reason!).

Circuit Training

Circuit training is a concept familiar to anybody who has been to a gym. It involves performing a series of exercises or activities (usually 6–10) in a certain order and with a set number of repetitions. The circuits are designed to avoid working the same muscle group in more than one activity. This is an extremely versatile method of training as the circuits can be designed by the coach to suit the particular needs of the horse, the rider, or the demands of the sport. Table 3.12 suggests a number

Table 3.12. Useful exercises for circuit training.

Exercise	Number of repetitions
Trot up hill, walk back down.	Twice on both reins
Trot up and down hill, maintaining rhythm throughout.	Twice on both reins
Lengthen the trot up hill, shorten the trot downhill.	Twice on both reins
Canter up hill, walk back.	Twice on both reins
Canter up and down hill, maintaining rhythm throughout.	Twice on both reins
Lengthen canter up hill, rider in forward seat; canter down hill, rider takes weight back.	Twice on both reins
Work over a pole on a 20-m circle.	Three circles in walk on both reins Three circles in trot on both reins Three circles in canter on both reins
Work over a small jump on a 20-m circle.	Three circles in trot on both reins Three circles in canter on both reins
Lay three poles out in a line 10 m apart; ride one-half 10-m circle over the poles.	Go down the line and back again twice in walk. Go down the line and back again twice in trot.
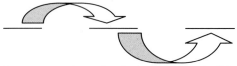	
Five trotting poles with pole 2 and 3 raised off the ground	Trot through three times on both reins.
Two poles placed a distance apart (avoid pacing out the striding too accurately, but aim for approximately four to six normal strides, five to seven short strides, and three to five longer strides)	Canter through twice on a normal stride. Canter through twice on shortened stride. Canter through twice on a lengthened stride.
Use four cones or markers to mark out a 20 m × 40 m arena. Leg yield in trot across the arena to change the rein.	Repeat twice on each rein.
Use four cones or markers to mark out a 20 m × 40 m arena. Lengthen up the long side, shorten along the short side.	Repeat twice in trot on both reins. Repeat twice in canter on both reins.
Work on a 20-m circle, at the same point on each circle do a downward transition to either halt, walk, or trot.	Repeat three times on both reins in walk, trot, and canter.

of exercises that can be used for circuit training in a field or arena. Ideally, coaches should intersperse canter exercises with trot and walk exercises and ensure the horse and rider have completed a thorough warm-up before attempting any of the exercises on the circuit.

Flexibility Training

Flexibility training aims to improve and extend the range of movement at a joint. A variety of exercises can be used, including static stretching, active stretching, and proprioceptive neuromuscular facilitation (PNF) stretching. Static stretching extends

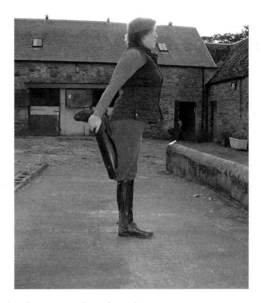

Figure 3.7   Example of static stretching for riders.

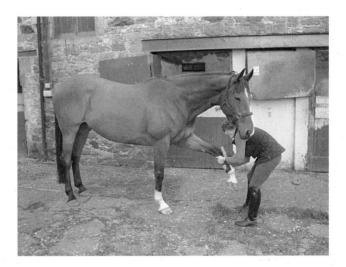

Figure 3.8   Example of static stretching for horses.

the limb beyond the normal range and holds it for 10 seconds from a still position (Figures 3.7 and 3.8). Active stretching involves movement. For riders it means extending a limb beyond its normal range of motion, and rather than holding, repeating this stretch rhythmically over a period of 20 seconds (avoiding bobbing or bouncing). For horses, typical exercises include lunging over poles, leg yielding, or working in brief periods long and low.

Training Programmes

Training is a systematic process designed to prepare horse and rider for the demands of competition. All athletes (human or equine) need to develop some form of training programme to prepare for their chosen sport. However, the type of training undertaken will vary depending on the discipline and the needs of each individual horse and rider. For instance, the impact of fitness is greater in the less technical and less complex disciplines than in those that require intricate or complicated movement. In other words, the impact of fitness is lower in disciplines such as dressage and higher in disciplines such as endurance and racing (Marlin and Nankervis, 2002).

The main principles to be aware of when developing a training programme can be summarised in the mnemonics SPORRT (specific, progressive, overload, reversibility, recovery, and tedium) and FITT (frequency, intensity, time, and type).

The SPORRT principle encompasses the general rules of training programmes (Table 3.13). They should be specific, progressively overload the body, provide time for the body to recover and adapt, be performed with the knowledge that fitness is reversible (any missed training due to illness or injury will result in the need to go back a step or two in the training programme), and be varied to prevent boredom.

Specific

In order for the training to be specific, the demands of the discipline need to be identified as well as the individual strengths and weaknesses of both the horse and

Table 3.13   SPORRT principle.

Specific	The demands of the discipline should be identified, as well as the individual strengths and weaknesses of both horse and rider to enable a sport- and individual-specific training programme to be implemented.
Progressive	For the body to adapt to overload, training must be progressive.
Overload	In order to improve fitness, the body must continue to be overloaded (in a progressive way) to produce a response.
Reversibility	Training adaptations are reversible. If training is stopped or reduced due to lack of time available or injury, then the body will lose the physical qualities it had gained through training.
Recovery	The body needs time to recover and adapt to overloading before it is overloaded again. If this is not done, then injury due to fatigue can be the result. Coaches should be on the lookout for the symptoms of overtraining.
Tedium	Variety maintains interest and motivation whilst avoiding boredom, staleness, and overuse injuries.

rider. These demands will be health and skill related. Sport-specific training means reproducing the demands of the competition within training but at a reduced duration, frequency, or intensity. For instance, preparing an endurance horse and rider for competition might involve training at low intensities (walk and trot) for prolonged periods of time, but not cover the same mileage as they would in competition. Event riders might train over smaller versions of the typical fences they will encounter in competition.

Progressive

For the body to adapt, the training must be progressive. If the body is suddenly given high training loads, it is unable to adapt and breaks down. The training programme should aim to start gently and build over a significant period of time. Equally, it is important to bear in mind that the cardiovascular and muscular systems respond rapidly to training, but the supporting structures (bones, ligaments, and tendons) take many months to adapt. In practical terms this means that although the horse (or rider) feels fit and well, care should be taken to ensure sufficient time is given to the basic fittening work before commencing more strenuous training.

Overload

The principle of overload suggests that the body will adapt to the level of work it is being asked to do. If the horse and rider continue to exercise in the same way, at the same intensity, and for the same amount of time, the body will get to a certain level of fitness but no fitter. In order to increase the level of fitness, the body must continue to be overloaded to produce a response. This can be done by altering the frequency, intensity, time, or type of training (FITT principle).

Reversibility

All training adaptations are reversible. If training is stopped or reduced due to lack of time or injury, the body will lose the physical qualities it had gained through training. Interestingly, riders suffer a more rapid reversal of fitness than do horses. Therefore, long periods of inactivity should be avoided, and if the horse or rider is returning from injury, training should be started at a low level and gradually built back up to pre-injury levels.

Recovery

The body needs time to recover and adapt to overloading before it is overloaded again. If this is not done, then injury due to fatigue can be the result. A good indicator of insufficient rest time for the body to recover is the resting heart rate. If it is above normal, especially first thing in the morning, then it is highly likely that the body needs more recovery time. Other indicators include loss of weight, increases in minor illnesses and injuries, decreased appetite, and general depression and irritability. These symptoms of over-training are true for both the horse and the rider. In particular, the coach needs to monitor the highly motivated horse and rider for these symptoms as they are the most likely to push themselves beyond their ability to adapt.

Tedium

Varying the training programme and methods of training helps to maintain interest and motivation whilst avoiding boredom or staleness. Also performing different types of exercise on successive days helps to reduce the risk of overloading and overuse injuries.

Structure of a Training Programme

All training programmes consist of general and specific elements. The initial fitten-ing work for all horses, whatever discipline they are competing in, is often termed long, slow, distance work (general). This is then followed by high-intensity work (sport specific) and skills training (sport specific). High-intensity work can refer to fast work, such as galloping, or strength work, such as working on steep gradients and gymnastic jumping. Skills training may include supplying exercises performed actively (e.g., ridden or ground schooling) or passively (e.g., stretching).

The training of human athletes follows the same structure, with individuals undertaking basic fitness work followed by sport-specific conditioning. For example, event riders require their training programme to deliver high levels of cardiovas-cular fitness and muscular endurance (general) as well as opportunities to develop agility and reaction time (specific).

The FITT principle relates to the detail within the training programme (Table 3.14). Each fitness session should consider the frequency, intensity, time, and type of exercise. Case Study 3.5 shows how this principle can be related to the fitness training of the horse and the rider.

Table 3.14. FITT principle.

Frequency	How often will the exercise(s) be performed?
Intensity	At what level of intensity will the exercise(s) be performed: low, moderate, or high? As the level of intensity increases the volume (amount and quantity) should decrease. Low intensity = high volume Moderate intensity = moderate volume High intensity = low volume
Time	How much time will be spent on the exercise
Type	What type of exercise will be used, and at what element of fitness is it aimed?

Case Study 3.5

Subject: Horse and rider competing at novice level eventing

Horse

Frequency	Intensity	Time	Type
Week 1 3 days per week	Low (walk and slow trot)	20–30 minutes	CV: hacking
Week 2 4 days per week	Low (walk and slow trot)	30–60 minutes	CV: hacking
Week 3 5 days per week	Low (walk and slow trot)	60–90 minutes	CV: hacking
Week 4 4 days per week	Moderate (walk, trot and canter)	30–60 minutes	CV: hacking
Weeks 5–8 3 days per week	Moderate (walk, trot and canter)	30–60 minutes	CV: hacking
2 days per week	Moderate (walk, trot and canter)	20 minutes	Skill: flat work & introduce jumping

N.B. CV = cardiovascular

Rider

Frequency	Intensity	Time	Type
Week 1–4 3 days per week	Low	20–30 minutes	CV: jog/swim/cycle
1 day per week	Low	20 minutes	Flexibility: yoga/Pilates
Week 5–8 3 days per week	Moderate	30–60 minutes	CV: jog/swim/cycle
2 days per week	Low	20 minutes	Flexibility: yoga/Pilates
1 day per week	Moderate	20–30 minutes	Strength: weights

SUMMARY

- Most riders will have a preferred learning style (activist, reflector, theorist, pragmatist) and will require a different coaching approach to optimise learning.
- Coaches should be aware that their own preferred learning style is likely to be reflected in their coaching style.
- Kolb's learning cycle suggests that in order for effective learning to take place, the rider must go through four stages: experiencing, reviewing, concluding, and planning.

- Individuals are likely to have a preferred informational style (auditory, visual, kinaesthetic, thinking), and coaches need to be able to vary their approach to giving information and instructions to accommodate these styles.
- Skill acquisition occurs in three phases: cognitive or thinking, associative or practicing, and autonomous or automatic.
- Physical fitness can be achieved in two areas: health related (cardiovascular, muscular strength and endurance, flexibility, and body composition) and skill related (balance, co-ordination, reaction time, speed and agility).
- The types of training available to the equine coach include continuous, interval, cross, fartlek, circuit, and flexibility.
- Training programmes include general elements and sport-specific elements and should follow the SPORRT and FITT principles.

Self Study

1. Consider the fitness demands (health and skill related) on both the horse and rider in either dressage, show jumping, or eventing.
2. Observe a number of coaching sessions and try to identify the learning and informational styles of the riders involved.
3. Devise a circuit-training session to include at least five different exercises (Appendix 5).
4. Design a training programme for a horse or rider using the SPORRT and FITT principles (Appendix 6).

Exam Style Questions

1. Discuss how coaches can use the knowledge of learning and informational styles to inform their coaching practice. Give examples.
2. Explain how Kolb's learning cycle can be used to organise coaching practice.
3. Describe the principles of training and how they relate to the horse and rider.
4. Evaluate the different types of training methods available to the equine coach.

REFERENCES

Christina, R.W. and Corcos, D.M. (1988). *Coaches guide to teaching sport skills*. Champaign, IL: Human Kinetics.

Davis, B., Roscoe, J., Roscoe, D. and Bull, R. (2005). *Physical Education and the Study of Sport*. Edinburgh: Elsevier Mosby.

Devienne, M-F. and Guezennec, C-Y. (2000). Energy expenditure of horse riding. *European Journal of Applied Physiology*, 82, 499–503.

Fischman, M.G. and Oxendine, J.B. (2001). Motor skill learning for effective coaching and performance. In *Applied Sport Psychology: Personal Growth to Peak Performance* (edited by J.M. Williams), 13–28. California: Mayfield.

Gunning, L. and Graham, K. (1997). Changes in the heart rate response of horse riders during the cross country stage of an equestrian three day event. *Australian Sports Medicine Conference, 1997,* 148–149.

Honey, P. and Mumford, A. (1992) *The Manual of Learning Styles.* Berkshire: Peter Honey Publications Ltd.

Kolb, D.A. (1984). *Experiential Learning: Experience as the Source of Learning and Development.* Englewood Cliffs, NJ: Prentice-Hall.

Marlin, D and Nankervis, K. (2002). *Equine Exercise Physiology.* Oxford: Blackwell Science.

McCall, C.A. (1990). A review of learning behavior in horses and its application in horse training. *Journal of Animal Science, 68,* 75–81.

McCall, C.A., Salters, M.A. and Simpson, S.M. (1993). Relationship between number of conditioning trials and training session and avoidance learning in horses. *Applied Animal Behaviour Science, 36,* 291–299.

Meyers, M.C. (2006). Effect of equitation training on health and physical fitness of college females. *European Journal of Applied Physiology, 98,* 177–184.

Mills, D.S. (1998). Applying learning theory to the management of the horse: The difference between getting it right and getting it wrong. *Equine Clinical Behaviour, 27,* 44–48.

Moore, J.M., Timperio, A.F., Crawford, D.A., Burns, C.M. and Cameron-Smith, D. (2002). Weight management and weight loss strategies of professional jockeys. *International Journal of Sport, Nutrition and Exercise Metabolism, 12,* 1–13.

Raether, J., Sanders, M. and Antonio, J. (2000). Strength and conditioning for the rodeo athlete. *Strength and Conditioning Journal, 22,* 31–34.

Rubin, L., Oppergard, C. and Hintz, H.F. (1980). The effect of varying temporal distribution of conditioning trials on equine behaviour. *Journal of Animal Science, 50,* 1184–1187.

Sappington, B.K.F., McCall, C.A., Coleman, D.A., Kuhlers, D.L. and Lishak, R.S. (1997). A preliminary study of the relationship between discrimination reversal learning and performance tasks in yearling and 2-year-old horses. *Applied Animal Behaviour Science, 53,* 157–166.

Planning and Delivering Effective Coaching Sessions

Chapter Objective

To provide an overview of the health and safety issues associated with equine sports, discuss the different types of planning a coach will need to undertake, and introduce the process of monitoring and evaluating progress.

4.1   THE COACHING ENVIRONMENT

The environment in which coaching is to take place is an important consideration for coaches when planning coaching sessions. Account should be taken of the health and safety of riders, horses, and spectators, as well as child protection procedures and risk management of all the activities to be undertaken (Figure 4.1).

Coaches also need to be aware of their legal responsibilities with respect to the advice they give riders and the way they supervise and manage participation in riding activities. Any advice or guidance given should be appropriate and should not go beyond the coach's level of qualification or experience.

Health and Safety

The injury rate for riders is relatively low in comparison to other sports; however, the injuries that are sustained can be more severe. The vast majority of horse-related injuries are caused by falls (Figure 4.2), crushing injuries inflicted by the horse, and

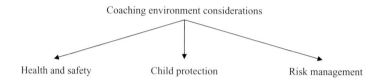

Figure 4.1   Coaching environment considerations.

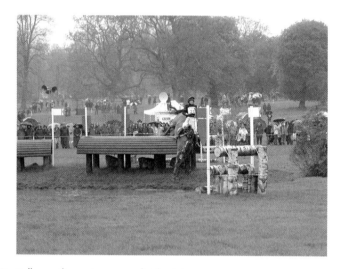

Figure 4.2   Falls are the main cause of rider injury.

kicks. Less severe injuries are predominantly bruises, cuts, abrasions, fractures (mainly to the arm), and joint sprains (Finch and Watt, 1996).

The largest group of injuries occur in the limbs and are mainly soft tissue injuries and long bone fractures. Head injuries are responsible for the majority of serious injuries and deaths in riders. Injuries to the thorax, abdomen, and pelvis are less frequent but are also often severe (McCory and Turner, 2005). Spinal injuries, although serious, are less common than head injuries and are most likely to be sustained during jumping cross country (Silver, 2002).

Research has shown that the major injury risk factors to the rider are from frightened horses, jumping, and ground conditions, as well as equipment problems and rider behaviour (Williams and Ashby, 1995). The main equipment problems are breakages of stirrups or girths, slipping of the saddle, incorrectly fitting footwear, and inappropriate rein lengths (e.g., adult length reins for a child rider). Rider behaviour relates to riding too fast, riding bareback, inexperience, and lack of concentration (Figure 4.3).

Coaches are responsible for the health and safety of the riders and horses in their charge. They must ensure that there is access to first aid facilities and the means to contact emergency services if necessary. A coach could be held liable if there is evidence that normal standards, practices, and procedures have not been followed.

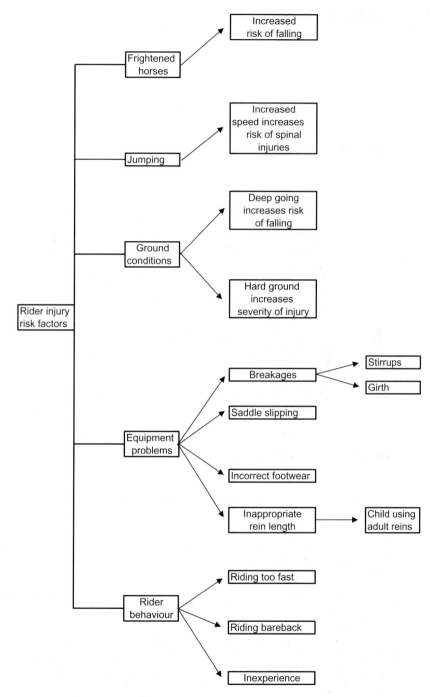

Figure 4.3 Rider injury risk factors.

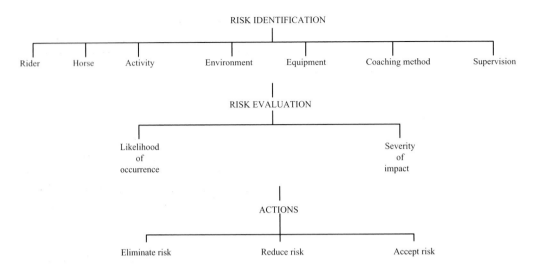

Figure 4.4   Risk assessment process.

At the start of the coaching session the health and safety rules should be explained to all participants. For instance when riding in an arena, riders should pass left to left; anybody in walk should keep to the inside track, with those in faster paces keeping to the outside track and avoiding riding fast up to or past others. There should always be at least a horse's length distance between the horse in front and the horse behind. Equipment should be checked for worn areas, insecure stitching, and poorly fitting or unsuitable tack. The rider's clothing and safety equipment should also be checked.

Risk Assessment

The objective of risk assessment is to produce the safest possible environment for horse and rider, and to do this coaches should undertake a risk assessment for each and every coaching session (Figure 4.4).

The first step in conducting a risk assessment is to identify the likely risks associated with the rider, the horse, the activity, the environment, the equipment, the coaching method, and the level of supervision.

The Rider

Consideration should be given to the general health and fitness of the rider, their experience and riding competence, their experience with the horse they are riding currently, and whether they are in the appropriate group for their ability and experience.

The Horse

Again, the health and fitness of the horse needs to be assessed as well as its experience, temperament, and the suitability for the rider. Clearly, if coaching at a riding school or similar establishment, it is much easier to match the most suitable horse with each rider. If riders are bringing their own horses, then the first job of the coach is to spend time assessing the suitability of that particular horse to the rider and adapting their session accordingly. A rider that is "overhorsed" may need to spend the majority of the coaching time developing control in order to safeguard their confidence and continued participation in riding.

The Activity

Clearly, some activities carry a greater risk of injury than others. Falls are more likely to happen when jumping, and the severity of injury will be increased as the pace of the work increases. Coaches must also reflect on the appropriateness of the activity in relation to the experience of both horse and rider, the suitability of the environment in which they are coaching, and the availability of equipment.

The Environment

The ground conditions, lighting, weather, and whether the area will be open or enclosed will affect the level of risk involved in a coaching session. A lunging exercise considered to be of low risk when performed in an indoor school may be considered unacceptable when executed in the middle of a muddy field in windy conditions. Although this may sound obvious, many accidents occur due to coaches using the same exercises when they teach in the indoor school for the riding club clinic as they do for the Pony Club rally in the middle of a field. Clearly, although the exercise may be a safe and appropriate one for the level and experience of rider and horse, the conditions in which it is to be performed may preclude it as an appropriate activity.

Equipment

In addition to checking the tack and clothing of the rider, all jumps, cups, poles, stands, cross country fences, dressage markers and boards, and gymkhana equipment should be checked to ensure they are appropriate and in good working order. Simple measures such as ensuring that jump cups are removed when not supporting poles; that fences are not sited where the ground is poor or has large holes; and that dressage boards have no protruding sharp edges, splinters, or spikes.

Coaching Method

The risk assessment also needs to consider how the horses and riders are to be organised for each exercise. When conducting a group session, will all exercises be carried out as a group, such as for flat work exercises, or will each individual take their turn separately, such as for jumping exercises? If working in a group, who will take the lead and who will bring up the rear of the ride? The coach must also determine that there is the correct progression of exercises to develop the skills of the riders and that these are appropriate for all horses and riders within the group.

Supervision

When planning group sessions, the coach should consider the number of riders within the group and whether there is a sufficient level of experienced help

Table 4.1. Risk assessment.

Risk Identification	Considerations
Rider	Health and fitness, experience, competence, experience with current horse, in appropriate group for level of experience and ability
Horse	Health and fitness, experience, temperament, suitability for rider
Activity	Appropriate for experience of horse and rider Conducted in an appropriate environment Appropriate equipment available
Environment	Ground conditions, enclosed or open, surface, weather conditions, lighting
Equipment	Condition and appropriateness of tack Appropriate clothing for rider All jumps – poles, cups and stands, cross country fences, dressage boards and markers, gymkhana equipment – appropriate and in good order
Coaching method	Riding exercises as a group or individuals, riding with or without stirrups, organisation of the group – lead horse etc. Correct progression of skills Appropriate for individuals and/or all riders in the group
Supervision	Appropriate ratio of riders to coach, sufficient experienced help available, appropriate level for child or adult riders, appropriate level of medical and veterinary cover, appropriate level of first aid cover and equipment
Risk Evaluation	
Likelihood of occurrence	Often – regular occurrence Infrequent – occasionally occurs Seldom – rarely occurs
Severity of impact	High – likelihood of severe injury Medium – potential to cause severe injury Low – unlikely to cause severe injury
Precautions and Actions	
Eliminate the risk	Remove the hazard (e.g., take unused jump cups off the stand) or don't engage in the activity (e.g., don't jump without stirrups).
Reduce the risk	Give safety instructions, provide repeated warnings (e.g., approach in trot; pass left shoulder to left shoulder; insist back protectors are worn).
Accept the risk	The occurrence is seldom – the risk is unlikely to occur. The impact is low – if it does occur, it is unlikely to cause severe injury.

Source: Martens (1997)

available. The ratio required is likely to be greater when the group comprises young children, inexperienced riders, or riders with a disability. In this area the level of medical cover, veterinary cover, and first aid equipment available should also be assessed.

The next step is to evaluate the likelihood of a risk occurring, if the occurrence could lead to an injury, and if so, how severe the injury is likely to be. Generally, a risk is classified as either a regular occurrence, an infrequent occurrence, or rarely occurs. The severity of impact is evaluated as either high (likelihood of severe injury), medium (potential to cause severe injury), or low (unlikely to cause severe injury).

Finally, the coach needs to identify the precautions or actions they will take to either eliminate, reduce, or accept the risk (Table 4.1).

Case Study 4.1

Karen developed a checklist as an efficient means of conducting a risk assessment for each of her coaching sessions.

Date:
Session type:
Venue:
No of riders:
Level:

Rider	Check experience – during introduction Check experience with current horse – introduction Check competence – observe warm-up
Horse	Check experience – during introduction Assess temperament – observe warm-up Assess suitability for rider – observe warm-up
Activity	Check equipment – on arrival Assess suitability of session plan – after warm-up
Environment	Check ground conditions and surface – on arrival Assess weather conditions or lighting – on arrival Assess suitability for session – on arrival
Equipment	Check poles, stands, cups – on arrival Check cross country fences – on arrival Check boards and markers – on arrival Check tack – during introduction Check appropriate clothing and equipment – during introduction
Coaching method	Assess suitability for all horses and riders – after warm-up
Supervision	Appropriate ratio of rider to coach – on arrival Appropriate medical and veterinary cover – on arrival Appropriate first aid cover – on arrival Appropriate first aid equipment – on arrival

Risk Evaluation

(For example)

Likelihood of a fall – infrequent
Impact – medium
Precaution/Action – acceptable if riders have appropriate hat, gloves, body
    protector, tack is appropriate and safe, and horse and rider are assessed as
    being sufficiently competent.

Grids will be jumped individually and no horses/riders to be left at either end
of the grid on their own.

Review Notes

(For example)

No incidences

In addition, all coaches should have an insurance policy covering public liability
and personal accident as well as a current first aid certificate. It is the responsibility
of the coach to find out if they are insured or need to arrange their own insurance
as well as what activities they are insured for and any special considerations or
exclusions. If they are coaching on behalf of somebody else, an organisation such
as the Pony Club or at an equestrian facility, they may be covered by the organisation's insurance.

A record should be kept of any accident that occurs, no matter how small. Details
of the date, time, place, name of rider, name of horse, activity, the nature of the
injury, a simple description of what happened (possibly a sketch) and what action
was taken should be noted (Table 4.2).

Injuries

Injuries can be classified as accidental, overuse, or chronic (Figure 4.5). Accidental
injuries, as the name suggests, are those that happen unexpectedly. They can be
caused by internal or external forces. Strains, sprains, twists, or tears are examples
of accidental injuries caused by internal forces. They can occur as a result of not
warming up properly or by moving suddenly. External forces are those outside the
body and result in injuries sustained by falling off, getting hit or kicked by the
horse, or by getting banged by a jump flag. Dehydration, heat exhaustion, and
hypothermia are also caused by external forces – the environmental conditions.

Overuse injuries are caused by repeatedly using a part of the body over a long
period of time. These injuries produce heat, pain, and inflammation. Common
overuse injuries in the rider are back, knee, and ankle problems. For the horse, the
back, feet, and lower leg are all associated with overuse injuries.

Injuries become chronic when they are not given enough time to repair. If the
rider or horse continues to exercise or is given insufficient recovery time, the injury

Table 4.2. Accident report form.

Date:	Rider name:
Time:	Horse name:
Place:	Activity:
Nature of injury:	
What happened:	
Action taken:	

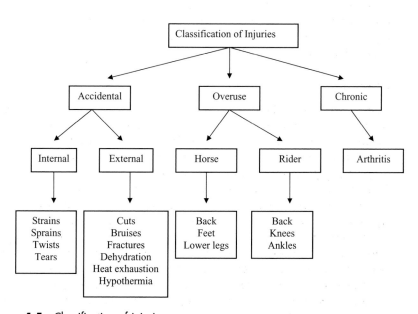

Figure 4.5 Classification of injuries.

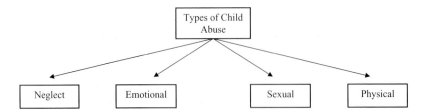

Figure 4.6 Types of child abuse.

takes longer to heal, and this delay can result in a chronic problem developing that can lead to permanent damage such as arthritis in the joints. The coach has a responsibility to ensure the horse and rider are fit enough and healthy enough to participate in the sessions and that they have had sufficient rehabilitation time following injury.

Child Protection

Each national governing body of sport is required to implement a child protection policy. It is the coach's responsibility to become familiar with the relevant documentation and act on its recommendations. By doing this coaches undertake to protect children from all forms of abuse and to take appropriate action if concerned about the welfare of an individual.

There are four main kinds of abuse: neglect, emotional abuse, sexual abuse, and physical abuse (Figure 4.6). Neglect occurs when a child's essential needs are not met. In sport neglect can take the form of exposure to extreme weather conditions, failure to seek medical attention for injuries, exposing a child to risk of injury through the use of unsafe practices or unsafe equipment, failure to undertake a proper risk assessment and therefore exposing a child to a potentially hazardous environment, and failure to provide adequate nutrition and water.

Emotional abuse is the failure to provide for a child's basic emotional needs. This can involve making a child feel worthless, inadequate, or not valued; imposing inappropriate expectations for a child's age or stage of development; and causing the child to feel frightened or in danger. A coach could be causing emotional abuse by persistently ignoring, humiliating, or being aggressive towards a child or acting in a way that is detrimental to a child's self-esteem.

Sexual abuse can take the form of inappropriate use of explicit language or jokes, showing pornographic material to a child, inappropriate touching, and sexual activity. Signs that a child may have experienced sexual abuse include lack of trust in adults, social isolation, low self-esteem, anxiety, depression, and discomfort or difficulty sitting and moving.

In sport, physical abuse is the actual physical injury to a child where the injury was inflicted or knowingly not prevented. This not only covers actually hitting or shaking a child but also failing to take action to protect a child from physical harm. Harm can be caused by overtraining, using unsafe practices or equipment, and failing to undertake risk assessments that take into account any physical limitations or pre-existing medical conditions.

Good practice when coaching children includes:

- Ensuring sessions are fun, enjoyable, and promote good sportsmanship.
- Treating all children equally with respect, dignity, and fairness.
- Keeping parents involved.
- Putting the welfare of the child first before winning or achieving goals.
- Being an excellent role model – avoid smoking, drinking, or using bad language when children are present.
- Being enthusiastic and giving positive, constructive feedback.
- Avoiding excessive training and competition.
- Recognising the individual development needs and capacity of each child.
- Providing a ratio of at least one adult to 10 children for those over the age of 8 and increasing this if younger children are involved.
- Finding out about any pre-existing medical conditions, injuries, and treatment.

Codes of Conduct

A code of conduct clearly defines what is acceptable behaviour and what is unacceptable behaviour on the part of a coach. It outlines standards of practice and helps to safeguard coaches by encouraging them to adhere to these practices. It also provides information for riders on what they should expect from a coach.

A code of conduct for equine coaches might include the following guidelines and value statements:

- Coaches must treat everyone equitably and sensitively regardless of gender, ethnic origin, cultural background, sexual orientation, religion, or political affiliation.
- The good coach is primarily concerned with the well-being, safety, protection, and future of the individual (horse and rider).
- There must be a balance between the development of performance and the social, emotional, intellectual, and physical needs of the individual.
- Individuals should be encouraged to accept responsibility for their own behaviour and performance in training; competition; domestic, academic, or business life; and in the case of the rider, for the health and welfare of their horse or pony.
- Coaches are responsible for setting and monitoring the boundaries between a working relationship and friendship with individuals. This is of particular importance when coaching young people.
- Where physical contact between a coach and rider is a necessary part of the coaching process, coaches must ensure that no action on their part could be misconstrued and that any national governing body guidelines are followed.
- Coaches should communicate and cooperate with other disciplines and allied professions in the best interests of the horse and rider.
- Coaches must not encourage riders to violate the rules of their sport.
- Coaches must never advocate or condone the use of prohibited drugs or other banned performance-enhancing substances.

- Coaches must ensure that the activities, training, and competition programmes they implement and advocate are appropriate for the age, maturity, experience, and ability of the rider and the horse.
- A key role of a coach is to prepare riders to respond to success and failure in a dignified manner.
- Coaches must accept responsibility for the conduct of their riders and discourage inappropriate behaviour in training, competition, and outside the equestrian arena.
- Coaches must consistently display high personal standards and project a favourable image of the sport and of coaching to riders, their parents and families, other coaches, officials, judges, spectators, the media, and the public.
- The coach has an obligation to project an image of health, cleanliness, and functional efficiency.
- Coaches must be able to recognise and accept when to refer individuals to other coaches.
- Coaches should regularly seek ways to increase their personal and professional development.
- Coaches should welcome evaluation of their work by colleagues and be able to account to individuals, employers, national governing bodies, and colleagues for what they do and why.

4.2 PLANNING SESSIONS

There are many types of plans that are commonly used in the sporting arena:

- Session plan
- Daily plan
- Weekly plan
- Monthly plan
- Yearly plan
- Competition plan
- Team plan

In equestrian sports, there will also be a plan for each horse to organise its training, development, and competition schedule.

Plans generally work towards a goal or objective and focus on:

- What needs to be done.
- How it needs to be done.
- Who needs to do it.
- Where it needs to be done.
- Why it needs to be done.

Yearly Plan

The yearly plan helps to ensure that there is enough time to develop the skills and strategies needed for the competition season ahead. It also helps to keep in mind what is important and what is a useful framework for evaluating the past season and developing a better plan for the next season.

The first step in preparing the yearly plan is information gathering:

- How many training sessions are there going to be?
- How many competitions are there?
- Are there any special events – qualifiers, demonstrations, camps, etc.
- How many horses are there and at what level are they?
- What facilities, equipment, and instructional aids are required and available?
- What extra support will be needed?
- What other factors might affect the yearly plan, for example, work and school commitments, holidays, team selection days, compulsory competitions, selection criteria, sponsor commitments, etc.

The second step in developing a yearly plan is to establish the goals of the year. This may involve an evaluation of where the rider is now, that is, their current knowledge and skills, a discussion about where they want to be, and also an evaluation of the previous year's performance. Once the goal(s) has been determined, the coach and rider should identify what needs to be done in order to achieve this goal. Each element is then broken down into smaller components and organised into a logical sequence of progressive coaching sessions.

To do this the yearly plan is divided into monthly, weekly, daily, and individual session plans, each with its own objectives (Figure 4.7). A monthly plan will include the objective for that month, any competitions that will be entered, and a indication of the number and nature of the coaching sessions to be undertaken. Weekly plans provide more detail about what is to be done during the week, including the number of coaching sessions and the objective of the week. Appendix 6 provides a template for a weekly training plan. Daily plans detail the tasks and coaching sessions to be conducted each day. This might include training for the horse and rider, fitness training for the rider off the horse, and any additional non-ridden sessions that the horse might require.

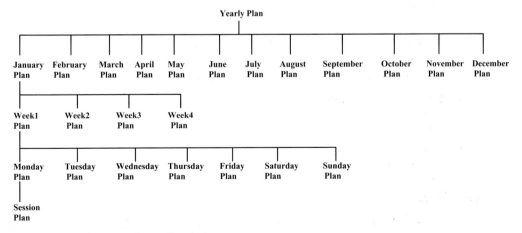

Figure 4.7 Planning – hierarchy of plans.

Individual Training Session Plan

Each individual coaching session should be considered as deliberate practice of a particular skill or exercise and therefore include a well-defined task of appropriate difficulty for the rider, feedback, and sufficient opportunity for repetition and correction of errors (Ericsson, 1996).

For competition riders increased importance must be placed on the development of competition-specific skills, and competition pressures and conditions should form an integral part of the practice setting to effectively prepare the horse and rider.

When coaching children, beginners, novices, or recreational riders, the activities should be broken down into small chunks of 5–10 minutes to allow riders to achieve success at a simple task and then progress to the next level.

A session plan contains the following information:

- Date
- Objective of the session
- The way in which learning will be assessed
- Prerequisites (e.g., fitness levels, experience, skills, knowledge, etc.)
- Equipment, facilities, resources required
- Description of the actual activities and exercises, including time allocated for each, key learning points, opportunities for feedback and discussion, and assessment activities and exercises
- Space for comments and evaluation: What went well and what could be done differently? Did the session meet its objectives?

Session Format

The actual coaching session is organised into several "chunks". The introduction is an opportunity for the coach and rider to set the focus for the session and discuss progress from the previous session. This is also the time for the coach to reiterate the health and safety rules, point out any potential risks the rider should be aware of, and confirm that both horse and rider are fit to participate.

The warm-up is generally 10–15 minutes long and designed to get the horse and rider ready to work. Clearly, the activities carried out in the warm-up will depend on the level of the horse and rider. For the beginner it might include simple exercises that can be performed on the horse, such as swinging the arms, circling the ankles, and stretching. The more experienced riders will generally have their own tried and tested warm-up routine for themselves and their horses. Whatever the approach, the principle remains the same – to raise body and muscle temperature. This means starting gently and gradually increasing the pace and flexibility required. Simple activities such as circles, changes of rein, and transitions between paces are effective warm-up exercises.

Following the warm-up is the chance to review what was done in the previous session. This is the rider's opportunity to show what they have learnt and practised and to demonstrate that they are ready to progress. It is the coach's opportunity to assess whether the rider is ready to move on or if more consolidation time is needed.

Once the coach is satisfied that the rider is ready to progress, the main exercise for the session is introduced and time given for repetition and correction of errors.

Ideally, this should last no longer than 20 minutes. The skill or exercise is described and, if possible, demonstrated. The coach picks out two or three key points to focus on and provides plenty of encouragement and positive feedback. The exercise may need to be modified to accommodate the progress being made or any problems that might be encountered. When coaching groups, the aim is to achieve full participation and improvement for all individuals.

The final activity is the opportunity to put what has been learnt into practice. This might involve riding a dressage test, jumping a course, or completing a series of movements. The aim is to put together a number of exercises that allows the coach to assess the learning that has taken place and for the riders to see the practical benefits of what they have learnt.

The end of the session is signified by a period of cooling down and stretching. The intensity of the activity is reduced, allowing the body and muscle temperature to fall and any buildup of lactic acid to be dissipated. The session should then be reviewed with the rider to indicate what they are taking away from the session. The coach summarises the objectives and key learning points and discusses the focus for the next session (Table 4.3).

Case Study 4.2 provides an example of a session plan (see Appendix 9).

Table 4.3.   Session format.

Introduction	Explain the format and purpose of the session.
	Explain what the riders should be aiming for.
	Explain any rules and health and safety considerations.
Warm-up	Raise body and muscle temperature.
	Start gently. Then increase the pace.
	Increase flexibility.
	Do simple activities, for example, circles and changes of rein, transitions, walk, trot, and canter.
Review previous learning	Since the sessions are progressive, this one should build on the previous one. As such, what was learnt previously is integral to the successful completion of this session.
Learn new skills	Describe the skill.
	Pick two to three coaching points to highlight learning aims.
	Provide plenty of positive feedback and encouragement.
	Full participation.
	Modify as riders improve.
Practice	Put together a number of elements such as movements in a dressage test or a course of jumps.
	This allows the coach to assess the learning that has taken place and allows the rider to see the benefit of what is being learnt.
Cool down	Decrease intensity of activities.
	Lower body and muscle temperature.
	Stretch.
Review	Review session – what was done and why.
	Identify key learning points.
	Prepare riders for next session.

Source: Robinson (2004)

Case Study 4.2

Date	*25 May*
Objective	*Be able to influence the canter striding between fences.*
Learning assessment	*Be able to ride between two fences on four, five, or six strides.*
Prerequisites	*Be able to shorten and lengthen the canter on the flat.* *Be able to count the strides between fences.*
Facilities	*All weather surface.*
Equipment and resources	*Minimum four stands, eight poles, and 12 cups.*
Activity introduction (5 minutes)	*Discuss progress since last session.* *Explain format and purpose to today's session.*
Warm-up (15 minutes)	*Walk, trot, canter on both reins.* *Turns and circles.* *Trot and canter over small cross pole with placing pole both reins.*
Review previous (10 minutes)	*Lengthen canter on the long side of the arena.* *Shorten canter on the short side of the arena.* *Grid work to count strides.*
Main activity (15 minutes)	*Upright to an oxer on comfortable five strides.* *Jump on both reins.* *Jump on five strides.* *Jump on four strides.* *Jump on six strides.* **Key points:** *Leg on and hold to shorten.* *Leg on and allow to travel for longer strides.*
Practice (10 minutes)	*Short course of related distances.* *Assess ability to influence the canter stride effectively.*
Review (5 minutes)	*Ask rider to reflect on learning.* *Summarise key points.* *Discuss focus for next session.*
Evaluation and comments	*Session went well, and the objective was achieved.* *Ideally, needed more jumps to make more challenging course to practice on – different types of fences – planks, double and treble and possibly go into the field and jump up and down hill.*

Schemes of Work

A scheme of work refers to a planned number of sessions over a fixed period of time to achieve a particular goal. For example:

- Pony Club summer camp working towards Pony Club tests at the end
- Group working towards BHS stage exams over a 6-month period
- Students at a college studying a module
- Intensive two-week course at an equestrian centre

As with all plans the first step is information gathering, as illustrated in Table 4.4. The coach needs to identify the rider or group dynamics – age, ability, experience, and the actual number in the group. Other information the coach requires includes: is there a set syllabus or performance criteria that the riders will be assessed against, what is it, and what needs to be covered in the time available? What form will the assessment will take, how many sessions are planned, and how long is each session? Are particular resources required, or does the coach have to work with existing resources? If so, what equipment and resources are available? Are theory, as well as practical sessions, required, and if so, how many of each type of session is required to cover the indicative content? How much revision and consolidation time will be built into the programme? What is the best order in which to cover topics? Will riders need to undertake any private study and practice?

This information is then organised into a table providing the coach with a detailed plan of what needs to be done and when (Table 4.5).

Table 4.4.   Information required to complete a scheme of work.

Rider and group dynamics	Age, ability, experience
	Number in the group
Is there a syllabus, performance criteria, module content to be followed?	What is the assessment criteria, learning objectives, or course content?
Form of assessment	How will the riders be assessed?
What time is available?	How many sessions will there be?
	How long will each session be?
What resources are required and available?	Do the riders need horses to be provided?
	Identify resources required for each session.
Balance of theory and practical	How many practical sessions
	How many theory sessions
What might need revision or consolidation?	How much of a review is needed at the start?
	How much revision or consolidation is needed during the session and at the end?
How should the topics be sequenced?	In what order should the sessions be run?
Is any private study or practice required?	Do the riders need to have time allocated to practice or for private study? If so, how much time and when should it be provided?

Table 4.5. Example scheme of work.

Scheme of work: Pony Club Camp (C+ group) **Group:** 6 x 14 year olds all passed C test
Syllabus: C+ Pony Club test sheet
Date: 1–9 July

Day	Time	Practical or Theory	Topic	Resources	Private Study and Practice
Day 1	AM – 1 hour	Practical	Mount and dismount Position at walk, trot, canter Increasing and decreasing pace Turns and circles Halt and salute	Grass, all weather arena	No
Day 1	PM – 1 hour	Theory	Stable kept pony	Feed, rugs, stable Bandages, first aid kit, grooming kit	Yes – read up chapter in manual
Day 2	AM – 1 hour	Practical	Show jumping	Show jumping course Grid	No
Day 2	PM – 1 hour	Theory	Foot and shoeing	Example of shoes Farrier tools	Yes – read up chapter in manual
Day 3	AM – 1 hour	Practical	Turns on forehand Sequence of legs in all paces Sitting trot and rising trot Walk on long and loose rein	Grass and all weather arena	Yes – read up sequence of legs in all paces
Day 3	PM – 1 hour	Theory	Fitting saddle and bridle Bits and their uses	Selection of bits Pony and tack	Yes – read up relevant chapter in manual
Day 4	AM – 1 hour	Practical	Riding up and down hills and banks Jump variety of fences and ditches	Cross country course	No
Day 4	PM – 1 hour	Theory	Grass kept pony	Rugs, grooming kit, first aid kit, feed	Yes – read up in manual
Day 5	AM	Practical	Mock C+ test	Arena, show jumps, cross country	No
Day 5	PM	Theory	Mock C+ test	As for theory sessions	No

Contingency Planning

With any plan there should be a contingency or "plan b". This does not need to be as detailed as the main plan but should consider what might happen and what action can be taken in response (Table 4.6). A contingency plan might identify the possible problems that could occur during the year and suggest other possible approaches, solutions, or courses of action. Alternatively, a contingency plan may be drawn up as a result of a problem or setback encountered.

Situations that may prompt the instigation of a contingency plan can include the horse or rider suffering an injury or a loss of confidence; a cancelled competition, a failed test or exam; or the rider not being selected for the team.

Coaches should always have a number of contingencies identified for their training sessions that identify what they will do if a rider fails to progress, the session

Table 4.6.   Contingency planning.

Possible Occurrence	Contingency
Horse suffers an injury.	Implement non-riding training programme. Receive coaching on a school master. Concentrate on another horse. Take opportunity to study for qualifications or attend clinics and lectures.
Rider suffers an injury.	Focus on psychological skills training. Take the opportunity to brush up on theory. Take the opportunity to get qualifications and attend clinics.
Horse and rider lose confidence.	Drop down a level. Take a break from competition. Plan additional training sessions. Temporarily get more experienced rider to train horse. Get some coaching on a school master.
Competition is cancelled.	Divert to another competition. Get in some more training. Change focus to next competition. Assess if competition objectives can be achieved in another way.
Rider is not selected for team	Find out why and what needs to be done to increase chances next time. Focus on another goal.
Test or exam is not passed.	Put plan in place to work on areas of weakness. Identify opportunities to get further training.
Session objective is not met.	Assess why and what to do differently next time. Assess if objective was realistic and appropriate. Assess what was achieved. Identify other exercises to help achieve the objective.
Rider is not ready to progress.	Select other exercises to work on. Repeat previous sessions. Take a different approach. Suggest areas for private practice.

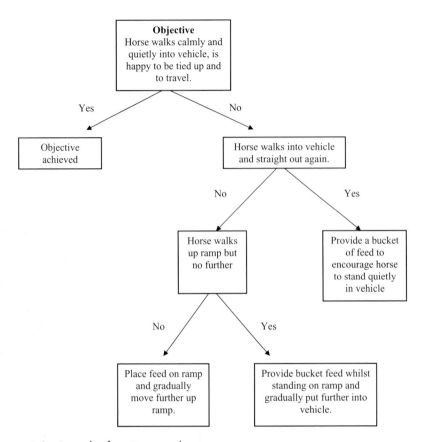

Figure 4.8 Example of contingency plan.

objective is not met, horse and rider struggle with a particular exercise, or the weather or equipment is not suitable.

Figure 4.8 outlines an example of a contingency plan that could be used when loading a horse into a horsebox or trailer.

Competition Plan

Each competition should have its own plan to identify the main objectives for both the rider and the horse. These may be to improve personal bests, use it as a confidence builder, or use it as a means of assessing progress or to achieve qualification. The clearer the objective for the competition, the easier the decision-making process on the day will be. For instance if the objective is to have a beginning of season confidence-giving run, rather than winning, then the decision as to whether or not to take the alternative route at a tricky combination on the cross country course can be made with less debate or deliberation.

Case Study 4.3

Competition	*Brook Farm affiliated dressage Prelim. 18*
Date	*10 June*
Venue	*Brook Farm Equestrian Centre*
Horse/Rider	*Jean Williams & Tosca*
Objective(s)	*Achieve a score between 62% and 65% (personal best = 64%). Ride all movements accurately to the marker. Achieve top 12 placing.*
Evaluation	*Got a score of 61.9%, which although below my objective, actually got me into 8th place. Good comments about my riding – got a 7. Good trot marks mainly 6s and 7s but only 5s for the canter work. I felt I rode accurately and didn't get any comments to suggest otherwise as I have on previous test sheets. The warm-up went well and I stuck to my planned warm-up routine. Felt very organised as I arrived early and had packed the car the night before so didn't feel as stressed as normal.*

Team Plan

Coaches involved with teams are likely to have a team plan. This might include a plan for selecting riders for the team and a plan for the competition once the team has been selected. These plans will include the competitions the team will be entered in, any warm-up competitions, when team selection will take place, the team riding order, and when and where team training sessions will happen.

Case Study 4.4

Team selection plan.

Team	The Shires Pony Club show jumping team
Main competition	Pony Club Championships
Date	25th August
Venue	Stoneleigh, Warwickshire
Objective(s)	Improve on last year's score of 16 penalties Finish in top 6

Short-listed riders	Claire Brown & Tom Cat
	Shaun Levy & Figgaro II
	Tim Hume & Clover
	Sara Hunter & Firelight
	Clara Smith & Jarmarama
	Pat Baker & Greyowl
	Sam Jones & Jasper
	Christopher Wright & Rialto
	Diane Wells & Lucky Lady
Team selection criteria	Consistently jumping double clears in 1-metre classes
	Experience jumping 1.05- and 1.10-metre classes
	Consistently reaching jump off this season in classes of 1 metre or over
	Top 5 finish in team trials
Team selection deadline	1st June
Team training details (dates and venues)	All to be held at Summerford Equestrian Centre
	5th June 6pm–7pm
	19th June 6pm–7pm
	3rd July 6pm–7pm
	17th July 6pm–7pm
	7th August 6pm–7pm
	18th August 6pm–7pm

Team Plan

Team	The Shires Pony Club show jumping A team
Competition	Pony Club Championships
Date	25th August
Venue	Stoneleigh, Warwickshire
Objective(s)	Improve on last year's team score of 24 penalties
	Finish in top 6
Team riders + reserve	Sara Hunter & Firelight
	Clara Smith & Jarmarama
	Pat Baker & Greyowl
	Christopher Wright & Rialto
	Diane Wells & Lucky Lady (reserve)

Name of Rider and Horse	Riding Order	Individual Objective(s)
Christopher Wright & Rialto	1	Two rounds scoring 0–4 penalties in each
Sara Hunter & Firelight	2	Two rounds scoring 0–4 penalties in each
Pat Baker & Greyowl	3	Two rounds scoring 0–4 penalties in each
Clara Smith & Jarmarama	4	Two rounds scoring 0–4 penalties in each

Team Tactics and Strategy

Both rounds all riders to go for safe clear rounds.
Best jump off horses – Rialto, Greyowl, and Jarmarama.
Team to be warmed up individually by own trainers.

All plans need to be assessed at their completion to identify their strengths (what went well and why), their weaknesses (what didn't go well and why), any opportunities to change and enhance the programme for the benefit of horse and rider (what could be done differently), and any threats that might prevent or may have prevented meeting the objectives.

4.3 MONITORING AND EVALUATING PROGRESS

Monitoring and evaluating progress is an essential process in three key areas:

* Identifying and correcting errors
* Checking that session objectives have been met
* Benchmarking

Identifying and Correcting Errors

One of the most common mistakes in coaching is to provide inaccurate feedback and advice on how to correct errors. This is often caused by rushing to make corrections before being certain of the reason for the error. It is better for coaches to continue to monitor what is happening until they are certain about why it is happening. As a general rule, the error should be repeated several times before the coach intervenes to correct it. This ensures that the error is something that requires attention rather than being just an uncharacteristic lapse.

Any errors that are observed need to be identified as either a performance error or a technical error. A performance error is when the coach knows that the rider is able to perform the skill or technique but for some reason is not performing it to the best of their ability. A technical error occurs when the rider has not learnt the skill or technique properly.

It is important to be able to distinguish between the two types of error in order to adopt the most appropriate approach to correction. When coaching beginners and novices, the coach's main role is to facilitate the learning of the skills and techniques needed to be able to ride. Therefore, any errors are likely to be technical in nature and require an approach that provides further detailed instruction and feedback to correct them.

Once the rider has progressed to the autonomous stage of learning, the individual takes increasing responsibility for evaluating their own progress and any errors are likely to be performance related. The coach still has a role to play in refining their skills and techniques, but the predominant focus shifts to helping the rider perform at their best. This may require encouragement to increase motivation and help with controlling anxiety or discipline-specific skills required to deliver a successful performance on competition day.

The associative stage of learning is the most difficult time for the coach to determine the most effective approach to correcting errors. It is likely that there will be a mixture of both technical and performance errors, and the coach will need to draw on their experience, judgment, and careful evaluation to decide the best way to tackle them.

When coaching more experienced riders, an environment where the evaluation of progress is controlled by the rider can be very effective. In this situation the coach delivers feedback only when requested by the rider. Research has shown that individuals in these types of self-controlled conditions require less feedback, demonstrate steeper learning curves, and perform better than individuals or groups using more coach-led methods of evaluation and feedback (Singer and Janelle, 1999).

Case Study 4.5

Anne coaches Sue, a dressage rider preparing to compete in the Advanced Medium regional finals. They have sessions once a month, and Sue usually arrives each time with a movement or series of movements she wants to work on or a problem or issue that she is having trouble resolving on her own.

For this session Sue asks Anne to have a look at the test she will be riding in the finals. In particular she is finding the canter half pass to flying change movements difficult. After warming up, Sue proceeds to ride through the test. At the end she mentions the half pass to flying change movement and says she thinks the problem is caused by the quarters trailing in the half pass. Anne agrees and suggests practising riding the canter half pass in medium canter to increase the engagement of the hind legs.

Sue practises this several times on both reins and then tries the movements in the test again. This time she feels it is better but is concerned that she may be blocking the flying change. She asks Anne what she thinks. Anne replies that she has noticed that Sue's inside hand is tending to come back during the flying change, and this may be preventing the hind leg from coming through. Sue rides through the movement again, this time concentrating on allowing the inside hand forward.

Checking Session Objectives Have Been Met

As discussed earlier in the chapter, the following questions can be used to plan individual coaching sessions:

- What should the riders be able to do at the end of the session?
- What activities and practise do they need to do to achieve that?
- How will they be able to demonstrate that they've achieved it?

Since the coach's primary role in these sessions is to facilitate learning through the use of objectives, instruction, and practise, the coach must take care to evaluate at the end of each session whether the planned learning has been achieved. Coaches are often tempted to judge the success of a session by how much they and the riders have enjoyed it. However, despite everyone having a good time, it is quite possible that no actual learning took place. This is why evaluating progress against objectives is so important. Clearly, the process of learning should be enjoyable for all involved, but success should not be judged solely on this criteria.

To encourage effective evaluation a fourth question to be answered at the end of the coaching session should be added: Can they do it?

If the coach can answer "yes" to this question, then (unless they have been coaching something the riders already knew how to do) the planned learning has taken place. If the answer is "no" for some or all of the riders, then the planned learning has not taken place irrespective of how good the coach's performance was or how much the riders enjoyed the session (Wallace, 2001).

Benchmarking

Benchmarking is the process of monitoring and evaluating performance against set standards. This can involve using external measures such as those set by an awarding body or internal measures set by the rider and coach (Table 4.7). The assessment criteria for Pony Club and Riding Club tests and BHS stage exams are examples of external measures. Team selection criteria, qualification criteria, and long-term rider development plans are also external measures. Internal measures that are set by the coach and rider include performance profiling, personal bests, and goal setting.

A benchmark identifies what the rider needs to be able to do at a certain level. For example, the BHS has very clear guidelines about what candidates looking to achieve their stage 4 riding qualification will be assessed on. This provides a useful framework for the coach to monitor and evaluate the rider's progress.

Experienced coaches have usually developed their own benchmark to determine when riders are ready to progress. For a coach in a riding school this might be when a rider is able to come off the lead rein or ride a more advanced horse. For a competition coach it might be when the riders are ready to move up a level or be put forward for team selection.

The fitness tests detailed in Chapter 3 provide benchmarks about what is an average score for each test. Riders can use this to judge their current level of fitness in a particular area and also to monitor their progress by repeating the test at regular intervals.

Personal bests can also be used to evaluate current performance against previous best performances. For instance, at the end of a season an event rider might look back and judge their success on having scored a personal best dressage score on

Table 4.7. Benchmarking.

External Measures	Internal Measures
Pony Club/Riding Club tests	Performance profiling
BHS stages	Personal bests
Team selection criteria	Goal setting
Qualification criteria	
Long-term rider development plans (see Chapter 5)	

their horse, achieved their highest placing at a particular level, or incurred their least number of penalties in the jumping phases.

Individual learning plans are a good way of monitoring and evaluating the progress of individual riders. They should contain key information on the characteristics of the rider, their riding experience, competition experience, fitness levels, aspirations, and current ability. Ideally, they should be completed by the rider in conjunction with the coach and should combine all the information gained through performance profiling, fitness testing, and psychological skills assessments.

Case Study 4.6

Name: Angela Smith	**Age:** 25
Height: 5'4"	**Weight:** 10 stone

Any limiting factors (medical issues/disabilities)	*Mild asthma – controlled with medication*
Riding experience	*Been riding since 7 years old, went to Pony Club, and has C test. Has passed BHS stage 3 riding and care. Owns 2 horses and participates in all disciplines.*
Competition experience	*Competed at elementary level dressage, pre-novice eventing, and newcomers show jumping.*
Fitness levels	*Needs to improve cardiovascular fitness. Flexibility and strength sufficient at this level.*
Aspirations	*Qualify for Novice Eventing championships*
Current Ability	
Riding position	*Generally balanced, secure, and straight. Tendency to drop left hip.*
Jumping position	*Generally secure and balanced. Tendency to look down over fences and be in front of the movement.*
Effectiveness on flat and over fences	*Able to influence horse well on the flat and over fences. Needs to develop discipline to be more accurate in transitions and approach to fences.*
Care of the horse	*Experienced and competent in the all-round care of horses in work.*
Training of the horse	*Able to produce well-mannered, disciplined, and enthusiastic horses to a good basic level of training.*
Psychological skills	*Good attention and concentration. Tendency to be affected by nerves during competition.*
Attitude	*Generally positive attitude, although a tendency to get down on herself when things are not going well.*
Strengths	*Hard working and intuitive rider. Good ability to focus attention and concentration. Enthusiastic and easy to coach.*
Areas for improvement	*Build on self-confidence as a buffer to anxiety. Ability to ride and train at a higher level. Improved discipline in accuracy of her riding.*

SUMMARY

- Coaches are responsible for the health and safety of the riders and horses in their charge. They must ensure there is access to first aid facilities, the means to contact emergency services, and have undertaken a full and detailed risk assessment.
- A risk assessment involves identifying the likely risks and evaluating these risks in terms of their likely occurrence and potential to cause serious injury. Precautions or actions are then taken to eliminate, reduce, or accept the risk.
- Coaches must ensure they have adequate insurance coverage and a first aid certificate, and that they record all accidents on an appropriate form.
- Injuries can be classified as accidental, overuse, or chronic, and are caused by internal or external forces.
- There are four main types of child abuse: neglect, emotional, sexual, and physical. A coach has the responsibility to implement the national governing body's child protection policy, to protect children from all forms of abuse, and to act on any concerns about a child's welfare.
- The coach should adhere to the guidelines and values outlined in the national governing body's code of conduct.
- There are many different plans used to organise coaching practice: yearly, monthly, weekly, daily, session, competition, team, and contingency plans.
- A session plan should detail the date, objective, learning assessment, prerequisites, facilities and equipment required, activities, and include space for reviewing and evaluating the session.
- There are three key areas where monitoring and evaluating is essential: identifying and correcting errors, checking that objectives have been met, and benchmarking.
- Individual learning plans can be used to monitor, evaluate, and record a rider's progress.

Self Study

1. Complete either a competition plan (Appendix 11) or a team plan (Appendix 12 and 13) for an individual or team that you coach.
2. Complete an individual learning plan for a rider you coach (Appendix 14).
3. Plan an individual coaching session (Appendix 9).
4. Conduct a risk assessment of the coaching session (Appendix 7).

Exam Style Questions

1. Describe the three main steps in conducting a risk assessment.
2. Explain the different types of plan a coach might use.
3. Analyse the importance of benchmarking in the planning and delivering of effective coaching sessions.
4. Discuss what should be included in either a good practice policy for coaching children or a code of conduct for equine coaches.

REFERENCES

Ericsson, K.A. (1996). The acquisition of expert performance: An introduction to some of the issues. In *The road to excellence: The acquisition of expert performance in the arts and sciences, sports and games* (edited by K.A. Ericsson), 1–50. NJ: Erlbaum.

Finch, C. and Watt, G. (1996). Locking the stable door: Preventing equestrian injuries. *Sports Medicine*, 22, 187–197.

Martens, R. (1997). *Successful Coaching*. Champaign, IL: Human Kinetics.

McCory, P. and Turner, M. (2005). Equestrian injuries. In *Epidemiology of Pediatric Sports Injuries: Individual Sports (Medicine and Sports Science)* (edited by D.J. Caine and N. Maffulli), 8–17. Basel: Karger.

Robinson, L. (2004). New Coach Education – Principles of Coaching Pack. *www.coachesinfo.com*. Accessed 31/05/07.

Silver, J.R. (2002). Spinal injuries resulting from horse riding accidents. *Spinal Cord*, 40, 264–271.

Singer, R.N. and Janelle, C.M. (1999). Determining sport expertise: From genes to supremes. *International Journal of Sport Psychology*, 30, 117–150.

Wallace, S. (2001). *Teaching and Supporting Learning in Further Education*. Exeter: Learning Matters Ltd.

Williams, F. and Ashby, K. (1995). Horse related injuries. *Hazard*, 23, 1–16.

Developing a Coaching Programme 5

Chapter Objective

To provide an insight into the long-term development of the rider, the use of periodisation in equine sports, and an introduction to performance analysis.

5.1   LONG-TERM RIDER DEVELOPMENT

Research has shown that in order for athletes to progress to the elite level of their sport they must undertake 10,000 hours of deliberate practice. This equates to approximately three hours of practice per day for 10 years, and it is known as the 10 year rule (Singer and Janelle, 1999).

In light of this, most sports have recognised the need for a long-term athlete development programme (LTAD). The majority of these programmes are based on a generic model with five basic stages (Table 5.1):

- Learning fundamentals
- Learning to train
- Training to train
- Training to compete
- Training to win

The fundamentals stage is aimed at individuals in their first three years of training. These are usually children between the ages of 6 and 13. It focuses on fun, basic

Table 5.1. Generic long-term athlete development model.

Stage	Emphasis	Training Year	Chronological Age
Fundamentals	Fun Basic fitness General movement skills	1–3	6–13 years old
Learning to train	Learn how to train Develop general skills	3–5	10–15 years old
Training to train	Event-specific training	5–7	13–17 years old
Training to compete	Correcting weaknesses Developing athletic abilities	7–9	15–19 years old
Training to win	Optimising performance	10+	18+ years of age

Source: Balyi (2001)

fitness, and general movement skills. Individuals should be involved in a number of sports to develop basic motor techniques of running, jumping, and throwing as well as experimenting with agility, balance, and coordination. A positive attitude to sport is actively encouraged, and activities should be chosen that allow children to feel successful, building confidence and concentration skills. The rules and ethics of sport are introduced as well as teamwork and interaction with others. Ideally, children should be undertaking these activities five to six times per week.

Stage 2 is learning to train, which involves developing general skills and learning how to train to become a better athlete. It is aimed at those in their third to fifth year in sport at an age between 10 and 15. During this phase, individuals are continuing to improve their agility, balance, and coordination through the use of fun games as well as beginning to undertake basic flexibility exercises, warm-ups, and stretches. There is a strong emphasis on skill development, and whilst individuals should be encouraged to participate in a variety of sports, this skill development will become increasingly sport specific. By this time there should be an understanding of the importance of practice and perseverance.

The next stage is training to train, which is directed at sport- and event-specific training for those in their fifth to seventh year in the sport (approximately 13–17 years old). Aerobic and strength training is a priority as well as flexibility and core stability. Sport-specific techniques are consolidated and individualised to address any areas requiring improvement. Formal mental preparation is introduced, with the emphasis on imagery, goal setting, relaxation, patience, and control. Individuals should be developing a sense of personal responsibility and discipline as well as positive communication and interpersonal skills. It is likely that individuals will be undertaking six to nine sport-specific training sessions per week.

Training to compete involves individuals in their seventh to ninth year in the sport who are likely to be aged between 15 and 19. The focus is on further developing athletic abilities and correcting weaknesses. This is a time of intensive training and optimum preparation for competition using tapering and peaking principles. Performance routines and pre-competition preparation are established as well as strategies for controlling anxiety. The individual is likely to be increasingly involved in the decision-making process and be developing the ability to plan, assess, and adapt to different situations. There is also an emphasis on increasing the knowledge base with regards to nutrition, hydration, environmental factors, and injury prevention and rehabilitation. This stage is characterised by 9–12 training sessions per week focusing on both fitness and technical and tactical skills.

The final stage is training to win. By this time athletes will be over 18 and have been involved in the sport for 10 years or more. This is a period of optimal performance. Training will have increased to 9–15 sessions per week focused on the maintenance and maximisation of performance, interspersed with planned periods of rest and recovery. Mental preparation techniques and routines are refined, and individuals are now able to make decisions independently based on both their knowledge and their experience.

The Equestrian Long Term Rider Development (LTRD) programme was introduced by the BEF in 2005. It aims to provide a structured approach to training children and teenagers from beginner to elite level in equestrian sport (Table 5.2). In contrast to the generic model, the equestrian plan has three main stages: learning and training to ride, riding and training to compete, and riding and training to win. These stages reflect the necessity of the rider not only to be an athlete in their own right but also to be a trainer and coach to their horses. They are also the areas directly relevant to the equine sports coach. There are a further two stages, Active Start and Active for Life, which relate to the early childhood period before becoming involved with horses and the later adult period when the focus for riding shifts to long-term career participation, for example, coaching, officiating, judging, etc.

Equestrianism is categorised as an early start, late specialisation sport. In other words, children should be learning to ride at a young age but not specialising in a particular discipline until their mid-teens. Ideally, they should also continue to participate in other sporting activities such as gymnastics, athletics, swimming, and vaulting as well as riding (Figure 5.1). During this time children will be developing the core components of athleticism (agility, dynamic balance, coordination, spatial awareness, flexibility, and basic endurance).

Table 5.2. Equestrian Long Term Rider Development Programme.

Phase	Age	Focus	Aim
Learning and training to ride	6–12	Learning to care for equines	The developing rider
Riding and training to compete	12–16	Learning to train equines	The competent rider
Riding and training to win	16–21 21+	Training equines to win	The complete rider The complete competitor

Source: BEF (2005)

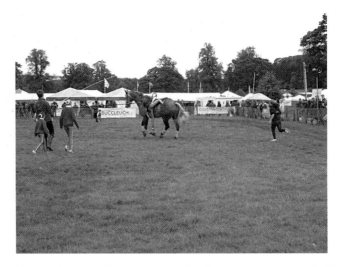

Figure 5.1   Vaulting is an excellent way to develop the core components of athleticism.

Learning and Training to Ride

This stage is aptly named "the developing rider". The ideal age range is 6–12 year olds, and the focus is on learning how to care for and ride horses in a fun and interesting environment. Coaches should aim to develop the basic riding skills of balance, feel, harmony, empathy, and control (start, stop, turn). Much of this training is done in riding schools and the Pony Club and should be multidisciplinary; that is, at this stage children should be encouraged to participate in all disciplines, thus developing versatility. The use of gymkhana games is an ideal way of developing these basic riding skills in a fun and enjoyable environment.

By the end of this stage the rider should be aiming to participate in low key competitions as an opportunity to experience the highs and lows associated with riding competitively (Figure 5.2). As a guide the split should be approximately 70% of the time spent training and 30% spent on competition or competition-specific training.

The coach's approach needs to be enthusiastic, positive, and encouraging. It should demonstrate and instil a love of the sport in a child- and family-centred manner. Gaining the commitment and enthusiasm of parents is crucial to the long-term participation of the individual. This is also the time to introduce the principles of discipline, a good work ethic, personal responsibility, and good sportsmanship.

Riding and Training to Compete

This stage is aimed at 12–16 year olds. By this time individuals should be developing into competent riders, and the focus shifts to learning to train horses. Coaches should be developing the skills of the rider in areas such as equine behaviour, physiology and development, and the refinement of their riding technique.

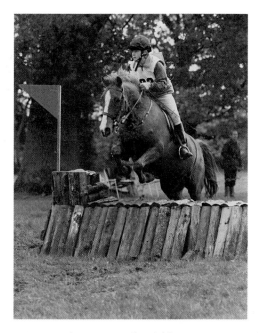

Figure 5.2 Competing is a good opportunity for children to experience the ups and downs of riding.

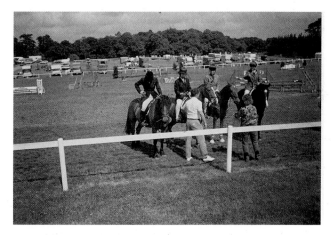

Figure 5.3 Training and competing as part of a team can prove a positive experience for young riders.

The main objective of this stage is the balanced development of riding and competitive skill. The split of training time is likely to be 60% spent training and 40% spent on competition or competition-specific training (Figure 5.3).

The coach's relationship with the rider should be developing into an adult-adult interaction characterised by mutual trust, respect, and collaboration. A balance needs to be achieved between pushing for excellence and providing unconditional support and encouragement.

Riding and Training to Win

The focus in this phase is training horses to win. It is split into two areas; the first is aimed at 16–21 year olds. At this stage coaches should continue to help refine riding technique as well as develop event-specific riding skills (Figure 5.4). The second area is aimed at 21 year olds and older and focuses on specific preparation for major competitions and the maintenance of performance at elite level (Figure 5.5).

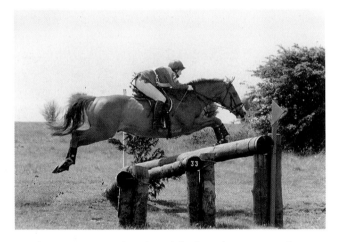

Figure 5.4   Developing event-specific riding skills through training and competition.

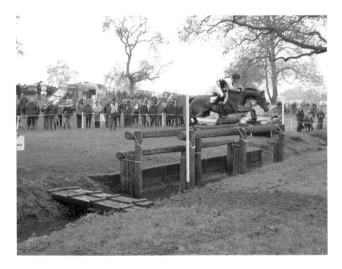

Figure 5.5   Competing at elite level.

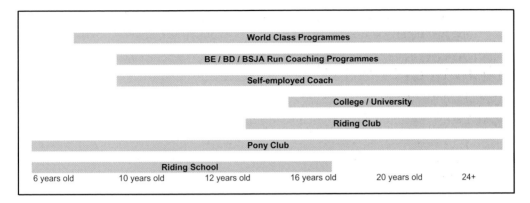

Figure 5.6   Potential sources of coaching throughout a rider's development.

By this time the rider is becoming an independent learner, and the coach increasingly becomes a mentor and sounding board, encouraging the individual to use their critical thinking skills and reflective practice to make decisions and solve training and competition problems. They are also likely to assist in the detailed planning of training and competition schedules and the analysis of performance.

Whilst the LTRD plan is predominantly designed as a tool to produce the next generation of elite riders, it can also be a useful framework for coaches to develop their own coaching programmes and used as a benchmark for evaluating the progress of the riders being coached.

In fact, it is unrealistic to expect that an individual rider will have the same coach from the time they start riding at 5 or 6 years old through to adulthood. It is more likely that they will receive coaching from a number of different coaches and through a variety of institutions and organisations (Figure 5.6). A typical rider might start in a riding school, progress through the Pony Club to a college, university, or riding club, and on into discipline-specific coaching programmes. In addition they may also have received discipline-specific coaching from a self-employed coach.

In order to ensure the most efficient and effective progression of riders through the levels of the LTRD programme to reach their potential, it is essential that all coaches use the programme as a guide for their coaching practice. This helps to ensure consistency in approach irrespective of where the coaching is being experienced. This means that at each of the three stages of the LTRD programme the coach should aim to develop individuals in the technical, mental, and physical skills required to ride effectively and successfully and not just teach riding technique.

5.2   PERIODISATION

Periodisation is a method of organising the training year into three periods – preparatory, competition, and transition – each building on the previous one but with its own specific aims and objectives. The preparatory period involves the general development of fitness and sport-specific skills. It may also include attending training competitions in order to fine-tune the horse and rider's performance.

The competition period is the main focus for the year and is geared around the important competitions such as championships or qualification for championships. The transition period is a time of active recovery in preparation for the start of the next season.

These periods are subdivided into a number of weeks called phases, each with its own objective for the development of the horse and rider (Table 5.3). The traditional model assumes there is only one main competitive season per year (a summer season) and has six phases, culminating in the main competition in August (Table 5.4 and Figure 5.7).

Table 5.3.   Phase objectives.

Phase	Objective
1 Preparation	Development of basic fitness and technique
2	Development of specific fitness and advanced technique
3 Competition	Competition practice
4	Refinement and preparation for main competition
5	Main competition period – achievement of goals
6 Transition	Active recovery and planning and preparation for next season

Table 5.4.   Single periodisation.

Phase	Duration	Months	Period
1	12 weeks	November–January	**Preparatory**
2	8 weeks	February and March	↓
3	8 weeks	April and May	**Competition**
4	8 weeks	June and July	↓
5	4 weeks	August	↓
6	8 weeks	September and October	**Transition**

Source: Dick (2002)

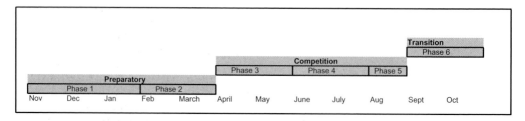

Figure 5.7   Single periodisation of a year.

Phase 1 lasts from November through January and constitutes the main preparatory period of 12 weeks. This is the time when basic fitness work is undertaken for both horse and rider. The objective is to develop cardiovascular fitness through long, slow distance work. Phase 2 comprises the final 8 weeks of the preparation period and focuses on the development of the discipline-specific fitness and skills required for competition. A number of training competitions may be included to obtain feedback on current performance and areas for improvement.

Phase 3 is the first of the competition phases. It is eight weeks long and extends from April through May. This phase is characterised by a return to serious competition but may involve starting at a lower level in order to build confidence and get horse and rider "match fit". Phase 4 is the eight weeks over June and July. As this is the second phase of the competition period, the coach should be looking for horse and rider to be progressing through the levels. The objective is a return to the standard achieved at the end of the previous season. The final phase, phase 5 is the main focus of the year and is the four weeks when the major competitions are staged.

The eight-week transition period of September and October is the active recovery and rest period for both horse and rider. It is an opportunity to reflect on the season's achievements and the progress made and to start to plan the following year's campaign.

Case Study 5.1

Sian and her coach have adapted the periods and phases of the single periodised year to plan their campaign in 2007, the goal of which is competing at the Novice Championships.

Season: Summer 2007
Event: BE Novice classes
Season objective: Novice Championships

Period	Phase	Duration	Months	Objective
Preparation	1	4 weeks	December	Basic fitness
Preparation	2	4 weeks	January	Flatwork and jumping
Preparation	3	4 weeks	February	Dressage and show jumping competitions
				Speed work
Competition	4	16 weeks	March–June	Pre-Novice and Novice events
	5	4 weeks	July	Prepare for Championships
				Step up to Intermediate and Open Novice
	6	4 weeks	August	Novice Championships
Transition	7	8 weeks	September–October	Wind down – one or two novice events for fun and gradually decrease work.
	8	4 weeks	November	Active rest – hacking out 2–3 days per week.

Each week of each phase will have an individual training plan that is then broken down further into daily training units. These training units provide the detailed information on the activities that will be undertaken each day.

If there is a winter season as well as a summer one, then a nine-phase model can be used. This system assumes that the climax of the winter season is in February/ March and the summer season is in September (Table 5.5 and Figure 5.8). The six weeks of November to mid-December become the winter preparatory period, followed by an eight-week competition period from mid-December through January, and into February for the winter championships. The six weeks from the end of February through March is the transition period between the winter and summer season. This is likely to be characterised by a period of light work rather than complete rest.

The summer season's preparatory period begins in April and concentrates on bringing fitness up to the pre-transition levels. Phase 2 constitutes the six weeks from May to mid-June, where sport-specific training is undertaken as well as a number of training competitions. The main competition phases, 3 and 4, comprise

Table 5.5. Double periodisation.

Phase	Duration	Months	Season
1	6 weeks	November and December	**Winter**
2	8 weeks	December, January and February	↓
3	6 weeks	February and March	
1	4 weeks	April	**Summer**
2	6 weeks	May and June	
3	5 weeks	June and July	
4	5 weeks	July and August	
5	4 weeks	September	
6	4 weeks	October	↓

Source: Dick (2002)

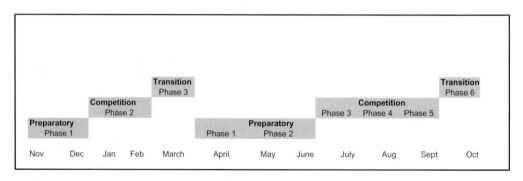

Figure 5.8 Double periodisation of a year.

five weeks through July and August, when a return to the competition levels of the previous season is achieved, and the four weeks of September, when the main competition and championships take place. The four-week transition period of rest, recovery, and reflection begins in October.

Case Study 5.2

David and his coach have adapted the periods and phases of the double peri-odised year to accommodate their plans for a winter campaign and a summer one.

Season: Winter 2007
Event: BD Elementary Dressage
Season objective: Winter Championships

Period	Phase	Duration	Months	Objective
Preparation	1	6 weeks	Nov & Dec	Basic fitness Flatwork schooling
Preparation	2	6 weeks	Dec & Jan	Strength training, for example, grid work and hill work Training competitions
Competition	2	4 weeks	Feb	Championships

Transition	3	4 weeks	March	Few medium tests for experience
				  and progression
				Active rest, recovery, and
				  reflection – hacking only

Season: Summer 2007
Event: BD Elementary Dressage
Season objective: Summer Championships

Period	Phase	Duration	Months	Objective
Preparation	1	4 weeks	April	Return to pre-transition fitness levels
Preparation	2	8 weeks	May & June	Flatwork schooling Strength exercises, for example, grid work and hill work Training competitions
Competition	3	8 weeks	July and August	Qualification competitions Medium tests
Competition	4	4 weeks	September	Championships
Transition	5	4 weeks	October	Active rest, recovery, and reflection – hacking only

Terminology

Much of the literature on periodisation refers to macrocycles (big cycle), meso-cycles (medium cycle), microcycles (small cycle), and training units. For ease of understanding, the terms *periods*, *phases*, *weekly training plans*, and *daily training plans* have been used instead.

Macrocycles = periods (preparation, competition, transition)
Mesocycles = phases (phase 1–6)
Microcycles = weekly training plans
Training units = daily training plan

The reason for consciously dividing the training year into these periods is to ensure variety in the training loads and skill demands of the horse and rider. A lack of variance can lead to both psychological and physiological problems, commonly known as overtraining or burnout.

Overtraining is a phenomenon most commonly found in highly motivated athletes who are most likely to avoid taking time for rest and recovery. This continual pushing of the body to its limits can have both physiological and psychological effects (Table 5.6). The individuals will notice symptoms such as prolonged muscle soreness that is slow to recover, general fatigue, frequent small and niggling injuries, and an increased resting heart rate. The outward psychological signs will be noticed by friends, family, and the coach. The individual will display increased levels of anxiety and stress and may be unable to sleep, look and sound depressed and irritable, and suffer from an uncharacteristic lack of motivation.

Peaking and Tapering

The purpose of organising the training year is to allow the horse and rider to reach the peak of their performance at the right time for the most important competition(s). In Case Study 5.1 this is the Novice Championships in August. Some horse and rider combinations may have several major competitions they are aiming for during the year. A dressage rider may have both the winter and summer finals, a show

Table 5.6.   Effects of overtraining.

Psychological Effects of Overtraining	Physiological Effects of Overtraining
Stress	Fatigue
Lack of motivation	Depletion of energy reserves
Increased anxiety	Muscle soreness
Depression	Injury
Unable to sleep	Increased resting heart rate
Irritability	

jumper may have Olympia in December and the Royal International in July, and an event rider might have Badminton in May and Burghley in September.

In order to achieve peak performance the volume and/or the intensity of exercise should be gradually reduced for the final 5–10 days before the main competition. This helps to preserve the mental and physical well-being of the athlete (be they horse or rider) and allow recovery of all the systems. It is contrary to the traditional "pipe opener" often given to event or race horses the day before a big competition.

The principle behind peaking and tapering relates to the process of completing the hard work required to achieve the necessary level of fitness for competition and then reducing the workload in the week leading up to the event, allowing the body and mind to recover and adapt. When exercising, small tears occur in the muscle fibres. These subsequently repair and become stronger as a result. In order for the horse and rider to be in optimal condition for the main competition, sufficient time needs to be given for the repair process to be completed. It also allows energy reserves to be replenished.

This process is equally relevant for the horse and rider. A rider who is riding five or six horses a day or working full time should consider reducing their workload in the run up to a big competition for exactly the same reasons. There are a variety of different ways that the work can be tapered in a discipline-specific manner (Table 5.7).

Table 5.7. Tapering examples.

Discipline	Examples of Tapering
Event horse	Replace speed work with hack Reduce intensity of work Jump smaller fences
Dressage horse	Reduce number of schooling sessions Replace schooling sessions with a hack Reduce level of intensity of schooling sessions Reduce level of difficulty of work in schooling sessions
Show jumper	Reduce height of fences Replace a jumping session with a hack or schooling session Reduce intensity of jumping and schooling sessions
Endurance horse	Reduce volume of work Reduce intensity of work Work at lower speeds Reduce distance covered
Polo	Reduce speed work Reduce intensity of work Replace with a hack or schooling session
Rider	Ride fewer horses Book time off work Reduce time spent doing other exercise

The event horse may have the speed work replaced with a hack or the general intensity of the work reduced by jumping smaller fences, working at a reduced pace, and doing less intensive schooling sessions.

The dressage horse may have their work tapered by reducing the number of schooling sessions – replacing them with hacking and reducing the difficulty of the work attempted in the school.

A show jumper might have the height of the fences reduced and schooling sessions replaced with hacking. The endurance horse is likely to have the volume of work reduced by decreasing the distance covered, and the intensity can be reduced by working at slower speeds.

Coaches may choose not to taper the workload for all competitions. In some cases, where the event is part of the preparation period and where the result is not of overriding importance, the event can simply be treated as part of the training programme. Equally, the coach may decide to taper the workload in training after a particularly intense phase of work to help maintain freshness and motivation in both the horse and the rider.

Strategic Layoffs

All riders should plan to have an annual period of active rest for themselves and their horses. This means that at the end of the season or between the summer and winter season there should be a period of quiet, relaxed exercise, two to three times per week. This is preferable to a complete break as it helps to maintain suppleness and basic fitness levels. It also prevents large fluctuations in fitness that can be detrimental to long-term soundness in the horse (Clayton, 1991).

It is not necessary for the coach to rigidly follow these periodisation models in their planning. However, it is important to implement the main principles: varying workloads to maintain physical and mental freshness, tapering to optimise performance, and a planned period of active rest, recovery, and reflection.

5.3   PERFORMANCE ANALYSIS

Observation is the traditional method employed by coaches to analyse an individual's performance. However, it does have its drawbacks. Research has shown that observations are both unreliable and inaccurate and that experienced coaches are more likely to detect differences between two performances (even when none existed) than novice coaches. They also tend to be very confident in their decisions, even when wrong (Hughes and Franks, 1997).

There are two main categories of performance to be analysed: the performance in the actual competition arena and the performance outside the arena, for example, the preparation and warm-up. One of the main reasons that observation falls short in terms of performance analysis is that it is often not structured enough to provide meaningful information. In order to combat this, the coach should identify and prioritise the key factors of successful performance. This provides the focus for the analysis and helps inform the decision-making process on the day of competition.

There are many different methods of analysing performance:

- Objective measures, for example, time taken, speed
- Subjective measures, for example, how it felt
- Observation, for example, what it looked like
- Questionnaires
- Videos
- Competition records
- Motion analysis

Some of these methods require expensive technical equipment that is beyond the means of most coaches, whilst others are simple but effective techniques that can provide valuable information for enhancing performance. For completeness, a brief summary of all the different methods and their uses has been included.

Objective Measures

Eventing is one of a number of disciplines where the speed at which the horse and rider are travelling can have a direct impact on the success of their performance. An optimum time is set for the cross country phase based on the stipulated speed and distance of the course (Table 5.8). Any competitors completing outside this time, or 15 seconds under the optimum time, incur penalties. These penalties could mean the difference between winning and not being placed.

Clearly, if a rider is incurring time penalties on the cross country course, then the coach needs to ascertain the reason for this. There are a number of possibilities:

- The alternative routes are being taken.
- Time is being wasted on the approach or departure from a fence.
- The horse is not travelling at the correct speed.

Often it is the case that riders, particularly those who have recently upgraded, are not aware of what riding at 520 metres per minute feels like. A simple way to analyse a rider's ability to judge the speed of their horse is for the coach to mark out a known distance and time the rider as they canter/gallop between them.

Table 5.8. Cross country distance and speed guidelines.

	Intro Pre-Novice	Novice	Intermediate	Advanced
Distance (metres)	1,600–2,800	1,600–2,800	2,400–3,620	3,250–4,000
Speed (metres per minute)	450	520	550	570

Source: BE (2006)

Case Study 5.3

Steven has been asked by an event rider he coaches to help get a feel for riding at 520 metres per minute. Armed with two cones and a stop watch, Steven marks out 520 metres around a field, and after a thorough warm-up, asks the rider to canter steadily between the points.

Ideally, if the horse and rider are travelling at 520 metres per minute, then it should take them 1 minute to travel between the two cones. On the first run they take just under 2 minutes. Next, Steven asks the rider to increase the speed of the canter – this time they are nearer to 1.5 minutes. On the third run, the rider is again asked to increase the speed and this time travels between the two cones in just over 1 minute.

After a brief rest, the exercise is repeated so the rider gets the opportunity to experience the feel of travelling at the required speed.

Steven suggests that this be practised once a week so that it becomes second nature for both the horse and rider to travel at this speed.

Subjective Measures

Subjective measures such as asking a rider how they felt the round went can be a useful source of immediate feedback. In Case Study 5.3 the coach could have taken the decision to go to a competition with the rider and at the end of the cross country course simply asked the rider how it went and if they felt they lost time anywhere. It might be that their horse was very strong and they found themselves constantly checking the pace to set up for the fences and changes of direction.

This type of questioning is also useful to uncover what the rider was thinking about or saying to themselves during the warm-up, prior to going into the arena, during the test or round, and then after finishing. The answers can provide an insight into the psychology of the rider at these times and may give clues as to why a particular outcome occurred. Research has shown, though, that free reports (unstructured discussion) of thoughts and emotions can result in many emotions and thoughts being added or omitted, particularly if there is a time delay, such as discussing the event with the coach at the next coaching session. A more structured approach can be achieved by using questionnaires (Tenenbaum et al., 2002).

Questionnaires

Most psychological research relies on the use of questionnaires (Table 5.9). The Competitive State Anxiety Inventory (CSAI-2) is used to assess an individual's level of anxiety at a given moment. It is designed to be used in the run up to and on the day of a competition to assess the levels of anxiety being experienced by a competitor and whether they view it as helping or hindering their performance.

The Sport Anxiety Scale measures the general levels of anxiety a rider might experience (trait anxiety) irrespective of whether they are at a competition or not. It also differentiates between the types of anxiety experienced – cognitive or somatic – and the level of concentration disruption caused.

Table 5.9. Sport psychology questionnaires.

Questionnaire	Author	Function
Competitive State Anxiety Inventory-2	Martens et al (1990)	Measures state anxiety – cognitive, somatic, and self-confidence
Sport Anxiety Scale	Smith et al (1990)	Measures trait anxiety – cognitive, somatic, and concentration disruption
Psychological Skills Inventory for Sports	Mahoney et al (1987)	Measures trait levels of anxiety, concentration, confidence, mental practice, motivation, and team focus
Task Ego Orientation in Sport Questionnaire	Duda and Nicholls (1992)	Measures trait levels of task and ego orientation
Profile of Mood States	McNair (1971)	Measures state levels of tension, depression, anger, vigour, fatigue, and confusion
Test of Attentional and Interpersonal Style	Nideffer (1976)	Measures trait attentional styles – broad internal, broad external, narrow internal, narrow external

The Psychological Skills Inventory for Sports identifies a number of psychological factors that could influence a rider's performance and provides the means for the coach to measure them. These inherent traits include anxiety, concentration, confidence, mental practice, motivation, and team focus.

The Task Ego Orientation in Sport Questionnaire looks at the trait levels of task and ego orientation. This information can allow the coach to make informed decisions about how best to motivate individual riders and also to raise their awareness of the potential pitfalls associated with the different orientations (see Chapter 2).

The Profile of Mood States measures the levels of tension, depression, anger, vigour, fatigue, and confusion experienced by riders. This is useful because when completed on a regular basis, it can help to identify problems or changes in how a rider is feeling before they manifest in poor performance.

The Test of Attentional and Interpersonal Style questionnaire helps to identify the predominant attention style of individual riders, for example, broad or narrow, internal or external (see Chapter 2). All these questionnaires can be used in one of two ways. The first is to profile the rider as to their strengths and the areas requiring improvement and subsequently to implement an appropriate training programme. The second is to use them as a diagnostic tool to establish why mistakes or poor performance might be occurring.

However, there are a number of potential downsides to the use of questionnaires, particularly for riders. Asking someone to complete a questionnaire just before going into the arena to perform is likely to mean dismounting, breaking concentration, disrupting the warm up routine, and possibly increasing anxiety by forcing the rider to think about anxiety and nerves.

Questionnaires are more objective than simply asking a rider how they did, and when worded well, can produce a useful insight into what is going on in their mind

(Tenenbaum et al., 2002). They also provide objective measures of psychological performance, allowing the coach to compare the results to benchmarked values.

Competition Records

Competition records can be a useful source of information on trends. Consider the dressage rider whose tests are marked subjectively and often by many different judges throughout the season. Individual marks on test sheets are unlikely to provide really useful information for the coach and rider as they are simply a snapshot on the day and reflect one mark for a movement that may involve several different actions (changes of direction, turns, circles, and transitions). However, it can be useful to analyse a number of test sheets to understand any general trends in the marks that may be affecting the overall placings.

Case Study 5.4

Neil coaches a dressage rider who competes at Elementary level. They are relatively successful, but seem to always be in the minor placings. Although the judges' comments on the sheets are helpful, there is no one thing that appears to be stopping them getting the marks necessary to win classes.

Neil suggests getting together all the test sheets for the last four months and doing some simple analysis on the scores awarded for the walk, trot, and canter. Ignoring the collective marks, they draw up a chart to record the marks from each test sheet and then calculate the average for each pace.

Walk	Trot	Canter
6	5	6
7	7	6
5	7	6
5	7	5
6	6	5
6	6	7
7	8	6
	6	7
	5	6
	5	5
	7	6
	7	7
Total =	Total =	Total =
Average =	Average =	Average =

Note: The chart contains only an example of the marks achieved as the full list was far too long for complete inclusion.

To calculate the total, simply add up the numbers in each column. To calculate the average score divide the total by the number of marks. For example, in the walk column the total is 42, and the average is 6 (42/7).

After completing this exercise, they were interested to find that the average score for the canter work was 6 and the average mark for the trot work was 7.5. As a result of this Neil decided their next few coaching sessions should focus predominantly on improving the canter to see if this would make the difference between a minor placing and winning the class.

Motion Analysis

Motion analysis is a method of using computers, video cameras, and sensors to analyse movement. Sophisticated equipment has been developed to allow many areas of the horse and rider interaction to be analysed, such as:

- Saddle fit to identify any pressure points
- Gait analysis of horses to assess lameness and its causes
- Shoeing and foot balance
- Rider technique
- Conformation and its relation to movement and lameness

Generally, this type of analysis involves attaching sensors or pressure pads to the horse, rider, or saddle. Whilst movements are ridden or fences jumped, information is fed to a number of cameras set up around the arena. The information can then be processed to produce three-dimensional representations of the horse and rider and then analysed using specialist software.

Motion analysis is likely to be beyond the scope of most coaches, although it is becoming more accessible to the general riding population. Some farriers, physiotherapists, and vets are already using it to help diagnose and treat injuries, and riders on the world class performance programmes are given the opportunity to experiment with it.

Observation

As previously discussed, although observation is the most widely used method of analysis in equine sports, research has shown that human memory is limited, and it is almost impossible to remember all the events that take place during a competition (or even a training session). Emotions and personal bias are also significant factors that can limit the quality of observations. The conclusion is that human memory and observation are not reliable enough to provide accurate and objective information (Franks and Miller, 1986).

Video

One of the most useful tools for analysing performance is the video camera. It is particularly useful because the "human eye" system is limited and events can be forgotten, distorted, or missed. The video provides a backup system for the coach and rider to support or refute any observations that may have been made during the competition.

Many competitors are in the habit of videoing their dressage test, show jumping round, or several fences on the cross country course. These tapes are then replayed at home to relive the experience and gain some insight into what went well and what could be improved upon. However, this recording generally does not give an account of what went on before the rider went into the arena or onto the course, that is, in the warm-up. Often it can be the peripheral things that have the greatest effect on performance:

- What the rider ate and drank
- What was said to the rider by coach, friends, family, other competitors, or officials
- What the rider was saying to themselves
- The length of the warm-up
- The quality of the warm-up
- The general organisation and planning of the day by the competitor
- What the rider did, for example, did the rider watch other competitors and did this help or hinder their confidence
- How the rider walked the course or learnt the test
- When they walked the course or learnt the test

It is possible for the coach to observe and make notes of all these factors without using a video camera. However, it is more powerful for the rider to be able to see for themselves the change in their body language, confidence levels, and self talk when they have, for example, watched other competitors in the same class. It is quite normal for individuals to be unaware of how they are affected by the things they do or say before they enter the arena. It is also quite normal for the rider to be adamant that they did not do, or say, or behave, or react in that way, so having visual evidence can help avoid a dispute!

Ultimately, the purpose of performance analysis and the role of video is to examine outcomes and the factors that influence those outcomes. An outcome relates to what happened when the fence was negotiated or the movement in the dressage test was executed. A successful outcome in show jumping means that the rider incurred no penalties at that fence. In dressage, an outcome is the score for each movement or the overall score for the test, and a successful outcome might be a personal best score, a placing, or winning the class.

To make the use of video more objective, a simple flowchart can be used to identify the actions, factors that influence the outcome, and provide a system for recording what actually happened – the outcome. For instance, in show jumping the coach might decide to look at the factors that influence the successful negotiation of a jump. These factors might include the turn to the fence and take off point, as illustrated in Figure 5.9. The turn to the fence is either off the right rein or the left rein. The take off point is either to the left of the jump, in the centre of the jump, or to the right of the jump (Figure 5.10). The jump is then recorded as being either successfully negotiated or unsuccessfully negotiated.

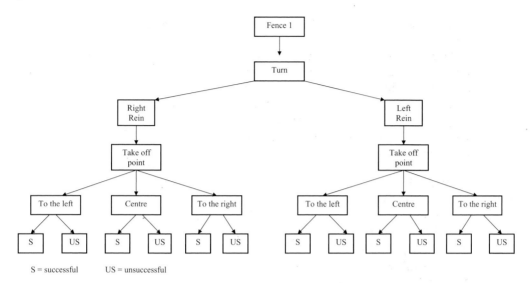

Figure 5.9   Simple flowchart.

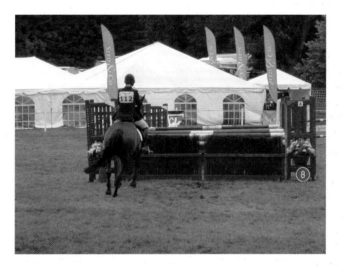

Figure 5.10   The take off point can be a useful factor to analyse in show jumping.

Once the possible actions have been identified, then the coach can devise a simple diagram to record the turn and approach to each fence in a course of show jumps (Figure 5.11). The true benefit of this type of analysis is when it is done over a series of show jumping courses so that trends can become apparent. Once a trend has been identified, the coach can either implement a coaching intervention to improve the likelihood of a successful negotiation of the fence or use it to inform the decision-making process.

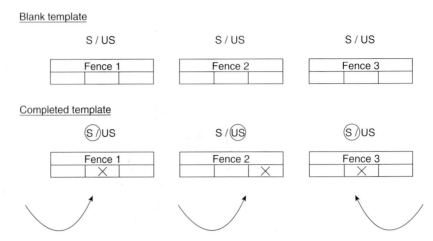

Figure 5.11 Show jumping template.

In the show jumping example, an analysis of a series of rounds might reveal that off the left rein, the horse and rider are twice as likely to have a fence down than off the right rein. Combined with the fact that the take off point on the left rein is more likely to be off centre than on the right rein, the coach might decide to implement exercises in the training sessions to work on improving the straightness off a left turn in order to increase the likelihood of the take off point being in the centre of the fence, and thus the likelihood of a successful negotiation of the fence. Alternatively, the coach may decide to use this information to advise the rider on the best strategy in the jump off rounds. In this case the coach might advise the rider to give themselves more room and time on the left rein to set the horse up and take a few more risks on the right rein where they appear less likely to knock a fence down.

There are other factors that could be analysed when show jumping (Figure 5.12):

- **Ground conditions:** Do the ground conditions affect the likelihood of the horse negotiating a fence successfully? If so, the coach might decide to conduct training sessions in different conditions to familiarise horse and rider with the conditions they find most challenging. Alternatively, this knowledge might simply help the decision about whether to use studs or not.
- **Types of fences:** Consider the different types of fences: doubles, trebles, planks, uprights, oxers, different types of combinations – for example, upright to spreads – and related distances. Is the likelihood of an unsuccessful negotiation of a fence increased for different types of fences?
- **Speed and time taken:** Does the speed of the canter affect the outcome of the round? A coach could measure the distance of the course and time taken to complete it to find the speed. If this is done over a number of rounds, is there any correlation between the speed and the successful negotiation of fences or,

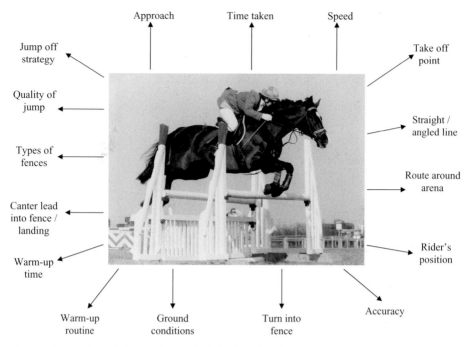

Approach   Time taken   Speed

Jump off strategy

Take off point

Quality of jump

Straight / angled line

Types of fences

Route around arena

Canter lead into fence / landing

Rider's position

Warm-up time

Warm-up routine   Ground conditions   Turn into fence   Accuracy

Figure 5.12   Potential areas for analysis in show jumping.

indeed, placing in the jump offs? What speeds are the winning horses and riders achieving?

- **Number of strides between fences taken round the whole course:** Is the route around the arena or the number of strides taken between fences influencing the outcome? Is the rider setting the horse up too much and therefore leaving themselves vulnerable to time faults, or are they cutting corners and distances, asking for longer strides, or taking "fliers" unnecessarily?
- **Canter lead into fence:** Does the canter lead influence the outcome of the fence being jumped? Are they more likely to have a fence down when on the left lead than the right? Does the horse land on one particular lead more than the other?
- **Warm-up time and routine:** When the rider has done well in a class, what warm-up routine was used and how long was the warm-up? How much time was spent in each pace, and how many and what type of jumps were used?
- **Rider's position:** Is there any correlation between the position of the rider's leg, upper body, head, and hands on the approach, over the fence, and on landing and the outcome at the fence?

The coach may also need or want to undertake separate analysis for the first round and jump off rounds, as they present different challenges for the horse and rider, as well as for the different types and formats of classes entered.

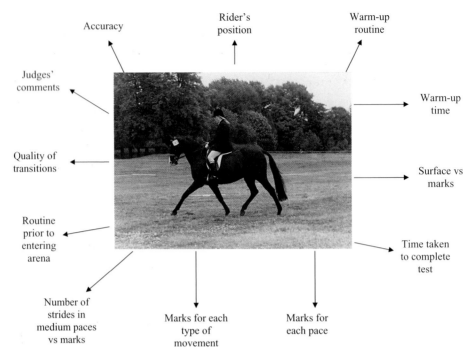

Figure 5.13   Potential areas for analysis in dressage.

In dressage the following factors that could influence the outcome of the test can be analysed (Figure 5.13):

- **Surface:** Looking over a season, is there any correlation between the surface being competed on and the marks awarded for each pace and movement? Does competing on the grass result in lower marks for the extended paces?
- **Time taken:** Each dressage test has a guide time given for completing it. Is the rider taking significantly more or less time to complete the test? Is there any relationship between time taken to complete the test and the overall mark? If the rider is consistently below the indicated time or the time taken by other competitors, could this indicate they are rushing through the test?
- **Marks for each pace or movement:** Are some paces or movements achieving higher marks than others? Is this consistent over a number of tests or over a season?
- **Number of strides in the medium, extended, collected paces:** Is there any correlation between the number of strides in these paces and the marks being awarded? Are those demonstrating more or fewer strides achieving higher marks?
- **Routine prior to entering the arena:** Is the same routine always followed? What is the variation in time spent going around the outside of the arena? If it is prolonged, does this affect the outcome of the performance? This can be important because it can help inform the coach and the rider's strategy. If a judge is holding riders for a relatively long time around the arena, a rider may choose

to take their time presenting themselves or alter what they do. Alternatively, if the judge is allowing them very little time around the arena, the rider may present themselves ready as the previous competitor is finishing to give themselves more time.

- **Warm-up routine and time:** How much time is taken in the warm-up overall, and does this affect the outcome of the test. How much time is spent in each pace, and what movements and transitions are performed? How much time is left between completing the warm-up and entering the arena? This might identify an optimum warm-up time and the most effective exercises to use to produce a high-scoring test. Figure 5.14 is a simple template for recording a dressage warm-up.

Rider & Horse: *Julie Brown / Adamant III*

Date: *16th June*   **Venue:**   *Brook Equestrian*

Level of test: *Novice*   **Test number:** *Novice 32*

Score: *65%*   **Placing:**   *5th*

Warm-up start time	10.05am	Warm-up finish time	10.45am	Total warm-up time	40 mins

Walk

Start Time	Finish Time	Movements Performed	Number of Minutes
10.05	10.11	Walk on long rein Circle 20m x2 each rein	6 mins
10.21	10.23	Walk on long rein around arena each rein	2 mins
10.40	10.45	Walk on long rein around arena each rein	5 mins
		Total time	**13 mins**

Trot

Start Time	Finish Time	Movements Performed	Number of Minutes
10.11	10.21	Around arena each rein Circle 20m x 2 left Circle 20m x 3 right Walk / trot transition x 4	10 mins
10.23	10.24	Circle 20m left	1 min
10.31	10.32	Circle 20m right	1 min
10.37	10.40	Around arena each rein	3 mins
		Total time	**15 mins**

Canter

Start Time	Finish Time	Movements Performed	Number of Minutes
10.24	10.31	Around arena Circle 20m Around arena	7 mins
10.32	10.37	Around arena Circle 20m Around arena	5 mins
		Total time	**12 mins**

Figure 5.14   Analysis of a dressage warm-up.

- **Accuracy:** Were the movements performed at the markers or accurately between the markers as required? Did the accuracy affect the individual marks for the movements or just the final marks for the rider? Is a good, but inaccurate transition rewarded with higher marks than a mediocre transition that is accurate?
- **Judge's comments:** If the comments are collated over a season, is there a trend of comments for a particular pace or movement? Do they give an insight into what a particular judge most values and therefore rewards?
- **Rider's position:** Does the position of the rider's head, upper body, leg, or hands differ or affect the pace or movement? Is the rider tending to be behind the movement in the extensions or in front of the movement in the trot to canter transitions? When this happens, does it affect the mark awarded?

It is often the case that dressage riders and coaches believe they have little control over the marks, as it is up to the individual, subjective views of the judge. However, by using performance analysis, strategies can be developed to ride the tests according to the qualities that particular judges value more highly than others. This is especially useful at the higher levels, where there are fewer judges and competitors are likely to encounter the same judges throughout the season.

If it can be identified that a judge forgives minor inaccuracies in favour of a high-quality transition, then the coach and rider know what to focus on. Equally, if a rider is consistently getting lower marks from a particular judge, they can analyse the comments and marks they receive, as well as those for horses and riders that are being well placed, to identify any differences in strategy or performance.

In addition to those factors already identified in show jumping, the coach could choose to analyse any of the following outcome-influencing factors for cross country (Figure 5.15):

- **Siting:** Is the fence being jumped uphill, downhill, in water, into water, out of water, into or out of woods, and does this affect the outcome?
- **Type of fence:** How many drop, skinny, double, related distance, bounce, step up, ditch, etc. are encountered? It can be useful to list the types of fences encountered during a season of competing as this will help to highlight the number and frequency of a type of fence to see if there is a subtle change in the questions being asked.
- **Time spent negotiating a fence:** How much time is wasted or gained when negotiating the fence? How does this compare to other competitors, particularly those who are close to or within the optimum time? Is the rider setting up too much or rushing the approach to try to save time? Are they kicking on after the fence or taking three to four strides to get going again?
- **Control and speed:** When does the rider start setting up for the fence, and how quickly does the horse respond? What is the speed of the canter coming into the fence, and is this due to rider choice or lack of control? Is the pace correct for the type and siting of the fence?

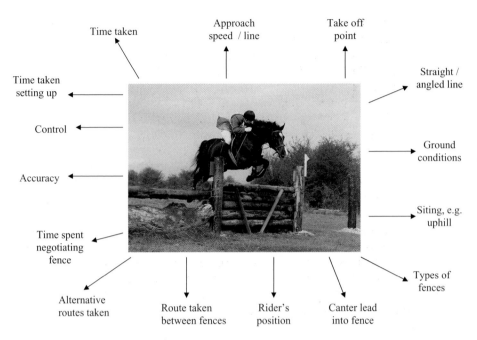

Time taken

Approach speed / line

Take off point

Time taken setting up

Straight / angled line

Control

Ground conditions

Accuracy

Siting, e.g. uphill

Time spent negotiating fence

Types of fences

Alternative routes taken

Route taken between fences

Rider's position

Canter lead into fence

Figure 5.15 Potential areas for analysis in cross country.

- **Accuracy:** Is the rider choosing a good line and sticking to it, or is it haphazard and reliant on quick reflexes? Did the rider stick to the plan, line, and strategy identified when walking the course?
- **Route taken between fences:** Is the rider taking the quickest route between fences or wasting time?

As always, it is important to relate these factors to the outcome of the fence (clear, stop, fall, stumble, hit the fence, run out, etc.), the overall penalties incurred, and the placing achieved.

Analysing an individual competition gives a record of what happened on that particular day and an insight into why it happened. However, the true benefit of performance analysis comes when a series of events or a full season is scrutinised to see if there is a trend or pattern of performance that can be replicated if it is successful or altered if it is hindering performance.

Alternatively, performance analysis can also be used to provide the coach and rider with information about how best to ride a particular dressage test, movement, show jumping course, cross country course, or fence.

An event rider might want to analyse the cross country rounds from Burghley to identify which alternative routes waste the most time and where time can be made up on the course. A show jumper might want to look at successful rides around the Hickstead Derby to assess the best way to approach the bank or the best line into the devil's dyke. The route taken by riders at a water jump (Figure 5.16)

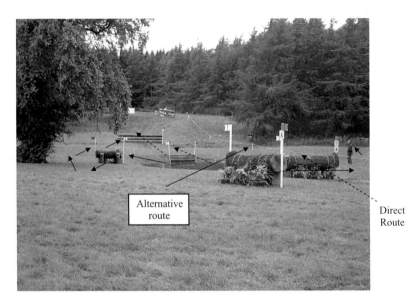

Figure 5.16 Routes at a water jump.

Competiton:	*Thirlestane Castle*	Date:	*August 2007*
Class:	*Novice*	No of competitors:	*32*
Fence:	*7 – water jump*		

Competitor	Direct Route	Alternative Route	Outcome	Time Taken
1	√		*Clear*	*1.30 mins*
2	√		*Stop at element A*	*2.45 mins*
3		√	*Clear*	*1.30 mins*
4		√	*Clear*	*1.35 mins*
5	√		*Stop at element B*	*3.01 mins*
6	√		*Clear*	*1.46 mins*

Figure 5.17 Template for analysing routes at a water jump.

on a cross country course can be assessed using a template such as that in Figure 5.17.

Dressage tests are now available on DVDs that show the marks given by each judge for each movement. A dressage rider could analyse the canter pirouettes of all the tests to determine which characteristics (size of circle, number of strides, regularity, tempo, and lowering of quarters, etc.) were displayed by the highest-scoring combinations.

The list of things that can be analysed is endless, and it is up to the coach and the rider to decide on what they specifically want to focus.

SUMMARY

- It takes 10,000 hours of deliberate practice to reach Elite level. This equates to approximately three hours practice per day for 10 years.
- The generic model of long-term athlete development involves five stages: fundamentals, learning to train, training to train, training to compete, and training to win.
- The BEF's Long Term Rider Development Programme has three main stages relevant to equine coaches: learning and training to ride, riding and training to compete, riding and training to win.
- Equestrianism is an early start, late specialisation sport. Children should begin riding at an early age, but not specialise in a discipline until their mid-teens.
- Periodisation is a method of organising the training year into three periods: preparation, competition, and transition. Each period is subdivided into phases, weekly training plans, and daily training units.
- Periodisation ensures variety in the training loads and skill demands of the horse and rider. It can help prevent the psychological and physical problems associated with overtraining.
- The traditional observation method of performance analysis is unreliable, inaccurate, and limited by the human memory and vision.
- The main purpose of performance analysis is to examine outcomes and the factors that influence those outcomes.
- Questionnaires can be used to analyse the psychological factors that affect performance.
- Competition records can be used to produce statistical information about competition performance.
- Video can be effectively used in all disciplines to examine individual performance in a single competition or series of competitions, or a class, or cohort of riders over a particular fence or course, or during a dressage test.
- It is important to analyse what happened before entering the arena (e.g., warm-up and preparation) as well as what happened in the arena.

Self Study

1. Design a periodisation programme for a horse and rider combination.
2. For three riders that you coach, write down the technical, mental, and physical skills you are aiming to develop as part of a long-term rider development programme. You should also identify which stage of the LTRD programme they are currently in.
3. Undertake performance analysis of:
   - an individual's show jumping rounds over a number of competitions (Appendix 15)

- an individual's dressage warm-up time and routine over a number of competitions (Appendix 16)
- the route taken by a class of competitors through a combination fence on a cross country course (Appendix 17)

Exam Style Questions:

1. Describe the stages of a long-term athlete development programme for equestrian sports.
2. Explain the benefits of tapering workloads prior to competition.
3. Identify three different methods of performance analysis and discuss how each can be used by the equestrian coach.

REFERENCES

Balyi, I. (2001). Sport system building and long-term athlete development in Canada – The situation and solutions. *Coaches Report*, 8, 25–28.

British Equestrian Foundation (BEF) (2005). Long Term Athlete Development for Equestrian Riders, Drivers and Vaulters. *www.bef.co.uk/Downloads/LTAD_Final_2.pdf*, accessed 24/07/07.

British Eventing (BE) (2006). *Rules and Members' Handbook.* Warwickshire: British Eventing.

Clayton, H. (1991). *Conditioning Sport Horses.* Mason: Sport Horse Publications.

Dick, F.W. (2002). *Sports Training Principles.* London: A&C Black.

Duda, J.L. and Nicholls, J.G. (1992). Dimensions of achievement motivation in schoolwork and sport. *Journal of Educational Sport Pscyhology*, 84, 1–10.

Franks, I.M. and Miller, G. (1986). Eyewitness testimony in sport. *Journal of Sport Behaviour*, 9, 39–45.

Hughes, M. and Franks, I.M. (1997). *Notational Analysis in Sport.* London: E&FN Spon.

Mahoney, M.J., Gabriel, T.J. and Perkins, T.S. (1987). Psychological skills and exceptional athletic performance. *The Sport Psychologist*, 1, 181–199.

Martens, R., Vealey, R.S. and Burton, D. (1990). *Competitive Anxiety in Sport.* Champaign, IL: Human Kinetics.

McNair, D.M., Lorr, M. and Droppelman, L.F. (1971). *Manual for the Profile of Mood States.* San Diego: Educational and Industrial Testing Service.

Nideffer, R.M.S. (1976). Test of attentional and interpersonal style. *Journal of Personality and Social Psychology*, 34, 394–404.

Singer, R.N. and Janelle, C.M. (1999). Determining sport expertise: From genes to supremes. *International Journal of Sport Psychology*, 30, 117–150.

Smith, R.E., Smoll, F.L. and Schutz, R.W. (1990). Measurement and correlates of sport-specific cognitive and somatic trait anxiety: The Sport Anxiety Scale. *Anxiety Research*, 2, 263–280.

Tenenbaum, G., Lloyd, M., Pretty, G. and Hanin, Y.L. (2002). Congruence of actual and retrospective reports of precompetition emotions in equestrians. *Journal of Sport and Exercise Psychology*, 24, 271–288.

Managing and Developing Personal Coaching Practice

Chapter Objective

To consider methods of analysing and reflecting on personal coaching practice in order to ensure continuing professional development through the use of action planning.

6.1   ANALYSING PERSONAL PRACTICE

Coaches are expected to understand and use an increasingly complex and specialised body of knowledge. Research suggests that the primary source of coaching knowledge is coaching experience. However, it is not just a question of the more coaching you do the better you get. Turning this coaching experience into coaching expertise requires reflection (Gilbert and Trudel, 1999).

A characteristic of effective coaches at all levels is continued ongoing learning and reflection. Reflection is at the heart of all experienced-based learning (Gilbert and Trudel, 2001). However, for this process to be effective the coach needs to gain adequate practical experience and ideally have a mentor or similar person with sound theoretical knowledge to support them. Otherwise reflection can remain superficial, and subsequent learning could be based on defective assumptions and inadequate reflections (Cushion, 2005).

There are many different methods of coach reflection, and each individual must find the method that works best for them:

- Discussion groups
- Mentoring

- Experiential learning
- Problem-based learning
- Keeping a reflective journal

The decision regarding which method(s) to use is likely to be influenced by a coach's preferred learning and informational style (see Chapter 3). An activist learning style lends itself to problem-based learning. Reflectors are likely to find keeping a reflective journal effective. Theorists may prefer discussion groups, and pragmatists are likely to get the most from experiential learning and discussion with a senior coach or mentor.

Discussion Groups

Discussion groups are made up of a group of coaches who get together on a regular basis to discuss coaching sessions they have run, any issues or problems they are experiencing in their coaching, or to share ideas.

Case Study 6.1

Jan and four other coaches currently studying for their coaching qualifications meet up on a monthly basis. They take it in turns to host discussion evenings, which usually involve drinks, nibbles, and lots of talking!

They each discuss the types of coaching sessions they have run in the last month, any sessions that went particularly well, any issues they had, and any good ideas or tips they have picked up. After this, they spend time discussing the coaching sessions they are going to be running in the next month, sharing ideas and exercises.

Sometimes they will invite a more experienced coach to these evenings to get their input or watch recordings of lecture demonstrations to get ideas.

Mentoring

Mentoring is a very useful system for all coaches, whether in training, newly qualified, or those who have been coaching for several years. Generally, it involves working with a more experienced coach to discuss ideas, talk through any problems or issues, and learn from their experiences.

Case Study 6.2

Mike works with a mentor who is a coach with many years of experience whom he respects and whose opinion he values.

When they first started working together, Mike used to talk through his coaching plans in detail, either on the phone or in person, to make sure there was nothing he had missed and to gain reassurance that he was going in the right direction. He also spent considerable time watching his mentor coach to pick up on good practice and how the varied situations that are encountered when coaching horses and riders can be handled.

As Mike gained more experience and confidence he asked his mentor to observe his coaching sessions and give him any suggestions or ideas for improving them and his coaching skills.

After several months, Mike began to ask his mentor for feedback on specific areas he had been working on or that he felt he needed to improve. Sometimes this was on the content or organisation of the session and other times it was on the way he conducted himself as a coach, the feedback and instructions he gave, and the amount of encouragement and positive reinforcement he gave.

Experiential Learning

Experiential learning can take many forms. It can involve doing as much coaching as possible at different levels and in different disciplines or it can be experiencing as many different types and styles of coaching as possible. In order to get the most from these experiences it is advisable to work alongside a more experienced coach or mentor who can highlight important or key learning points.

Case Study 6.3

Sarah found that the most effective way for her to learn about different styles of coaching was to actually experience it for herself. This approach allowed her to view the coaching from a participant's point of view and gave her really useful insights into what worked and what didn't.

To get as varied a coaching experience as possible she regularly attended training days run by the local equestrian centre and riding club. She also volunteered as a guinea pig rider for those taking their BHS teaching exams and in any lecture demonstrations in the area. If she was unable to ride, she made the effort to go along and watch.

After each of these experiences she wrote down any "top tips", any good exercises, and her thoughts about what she liked and didn't like about the session.

Problem-Based Learning

Problem-based learning is a technique often employed in theoretical training sessions. It involves setting a problem or scenario and asking the participants to suggest solutions to the problem or approaches to the situation. It is a useful method for reflecting on the different options available and their pros and cons.

Case Study 6.4

Chris and Lisa are newly qualified coaches who are gaining experience coaching at a college. They both trained and qualified together and found discussing coaching scenarios really useful when they were revising for their assessments.

They decided to keep this going once they were qualified, meeting on a regular basis to set each other coaching problems to work through. Sometimes this is something they have encountered in their coaching sessions, such as a rider who has lost confidence jumping or how to keep all the riders in a group flatwork session challenged. Other times they envision situations they might come across and possible ways to resolve them, such as a horse who won't go through the water on a cross country training session or a rider who loses balance and falls behind the movement when jumping.

For each scenario they discussed various options. If they found a problem or scenario they were unsure about or for which they were unable to suggest a suitable approach, they would investigate it further. This was done by talking to other coaches, reading books or magazine articles, or watching videos of lecture demonstrations or master classes.

Keeping a Reflective Journal

A reflective journal is used to log events, to describe circumstances, and to record and reflect upon incidents and experiences that will help develop and enhance professional practice (Wallace, 2001).

To ensure the journal moves beyond the purely descriptive, a coach can use questions to direct their thinking and reflection:

- What went well and why?
- What didn't go well and why?
- What am I going to do differently?
- What have I learnt about myself, my subject knowledge, my coaching skills, the riders and horses?
- Did I enjoy this session? Why?
- Did the riders seem to enjoy the session? Why?
- Were the learning objectives achieved? How?

It is not necessary to write pages and pages; the measure of a good reflective journal is that the individual is asking questions and then attempting to answer them. It should chart concerns, solutions, development or training needs, and successes, in other words it is charting and planning a coach's own professional development. If the journal is productive, it will generally end in action points or an entire plan of action (Wallace, 2001).

Case Study 6.5

Caroline found writing a reflective journal quite difficult so she devised a one-page template of questions that she attached to her session plan and risk assessment for each coaching session. She used this template to review each coaching session by answering the questions.

Session: Date:	
What went well and why?	
What didn't go well and why?	
What would I do differently?	
What have I learnt about: 1. myself 2. my subject knowledge 3. my coaching skills 4. the riders/horses	
How can I apply what I have learnt?	
What do I need to learn more about?	
What am I going to do next?	1. 2. 3.

Other areas a coach might want to consider when reflecting on their coaching sessions are listed below and detailed in Table 6.1:

- Health and safety
- Communication
- Session content, structure, and planning

Table 6.1. Areas of reflection.

Health and safety	Were the facilities and equipment checked for safety?
	Was a risk assessment carried out?
	Was the experience of horse and rider checked?
Content, structure, and planning	Was there a clear plan of work?
	Were there objectives for each session?
	Was there an appropriate warm up and cool down?
	Were the sessions and exercises progressive?
	Was there an assessment of what had been learned?
Communication	Were riders informed of the session content and objectives?
	Were riders checked for understanding?
	Were riders made aware of any rules or codes of conduct?
	Were instructions clear, concise, and appropriate?
	Was the coach's body language and tone of voice appropriate?
	Were explanations and demonstrations appropriate and clear?
Monitoring of riders	Was positive feedback given?
	Was appropriate corrective action provided?
	Were riders allowed to ask questions?
	Were appropriate coaching methods used to develop each rider?
	Were riders asked for feedback on the session?
	Were all riders given equal time and attention?
Knowledge and experience	Did the riders enjoy the session?
	Was it a positive experience for riders, horses, and coach?
	Did the coach show clear understanding of the techniques and skills?
	Did the riders respect and trust the coach?
	Did the coach analyse what worked well and what didn't and how to change it?

Source: Martens (1997)

- Knowledge and experience
- Monitoring and evaluating of riders

Ultimately, through a high level of subject knowledge, coaching expertise, and reflection, a coach should be aiming to achieve sessions that:

- Consistently challenge all riders
- Include activities that closely match the riders' development needs
- Promote independent learning
- Are thoroughly prepared
- Make effective use of unanticipated but productive opportunities that arise
- Inspire riders through the coach's enthusiasm and commitment
- Achieve progress that is considerably better than might be expected
- Provide effective feedback

6.2   PERSONAL ACTION PLANNING

Personal action planning is the process of asking and answering the questions, What kind of coaching career do I want? and What action do I need to take in order to get the career that I want?

The first step is for the coach to consider what they want their future career to be like.

- What type of coaching do they want to be involved in?
- Who do they want to be coaching?
- Where do they want to be coaching?
- Do they want to be employed by an organisation or work independently?

Case Study 6.6

Nicki decided that in five year's time she wanted to be the resident head coach in an equestrian centre, coaching competition riders of all ages and in all disciplines. She liked the idea of being based in one place and receiving a regular monthly salary as well as having access to high-quality facilities and horses. She also liked the idea of being able to share what she had learned by working with trainees and newly qualified coaches.

The next step is for the coach to consider their current situation. What skills, knowledge, and attributes do they currently possess that will help them to achieve their career goal.

Case Study 6.6 (cont.)

Having chosen her career goal, Nicki decided to undertake an audit to identify the coaching skills, knowledge, and experience she currently possessed, so she devised a template to collate all this information.

Coaching Skills	Communication	*I get on well with the riders I coach and the feedback I get is that they enjoy the lessons, understand what is being explained and are pleased with their progress.*
		I regularly use questions to check for understanding.
		I am careful to give instructions clearly and concisely.

	Planning	All my coaching sessions have a plan that includes an objective, warm-up, main activity, and cooldown exercises.
		I use a template to plan all the sessions and keep them for future reference.
	Feedback	I make sure there are opportunities for giving feedback to each rider in the session and always ensure the feedback is positive and useful.
		Each rider is given something to work on for the next session.
	Reflection	I always make time to evaluate each session.
Knowledge	Developing horses	I spent my work placement year at college working at an event yard where I was involved in backing young horses, fittening work on the older horses, and took my own horse with me to get help with training him to novice level.
		I have ridden trained and ridden horses to novice level eventing, medium level dressage and show jumped to Newcomer level.
	Developing riders	During my training for my coaching qualification I worked in a riding school for 2 years and have taught at Pony Club camp.
		I have the BHS AI qualification.
	Sports psychology	I have been interested in sport psychology through my own competing and have read books and practised exercises for reducing anxiety and using imagery.
	Horse behaviour	Whilst studying at college, I completed a module on equine behaviour.
Experience	Coaching children	I have quite a lot of experience (2–3 years) of coaching children ranging from 4 years old to 14 years old at a local riding school and a local Pony Club.
	Discipline-specific	I have competed in affiliated dressage, show jumping, and eventing.

The final step is for the coach to undertake further research to identify the skills, knowledge, and experience they will need in their chosen career. This can be done by looking through job advertisements, talking to individuals who are currently in the job, or talking to employers who are likely to be recruiting for the job.

Case Study 6.6 (cont.)

Nicki now decided to contact a coach who worked at the local equestrian centre. She telephoned the centre and spoke to the coach, who suggested she come in the next day.

When she arrived, she was surprised to find that the owner of the equestrian centre was also there and happy to talk about what was important to them when they were looking to employ a coach.

After the discussion, Nicki came away with a list of the knowledge and practical experience she needed to achieve her career goal:

- Experience coaching adults and children
- Experience coaching competition riders
- A level 3 coaching qualification (BHS, UKCC, or degree)
- Experience developing and implementing coaching programmes
- High level of knowledge in all aspects of coaching horses and riders
- Strong communication skills
- Strong organisation and planning skills
- A commitment to personal development
- A commitment to keeping up to date with current advances in coaching horses and riders

Once all this information has been gathered it can be collated in the form of a gap analysis. A gap analysis allows the coach to compare where they are now to where they want to be and identify ways to close the gap between the two. This might involve undertaking further study or work experience, attending seminars, or applying for jobs that have the scope to allow for personal development in relevant areas.

Profiling (Chapter 2) is an effective method of gap analysis, and it also helps to prioritise areas for development. The coach rates each area required for their chosen career according to its importance (on a scale of 1 to 10). Then each area is rated according to the coach's perceived competence in that area (again on a scale of 1 to 10). The bigger the gap between the two scores, the higher the priority this area should be given (Table 6.2).

When the profile has been completed, the coach should have a clearer idea about which areas need attention and in what order of priority. In Table 6.2, there are four areas that are rated as 10 out of 10 for importance but only 1 out of 10 on self-evaluation. These areas should be considered high priorities and form the basis of an action plan.

The Action Plan

An action plan is where the coach records what they intend to do, how they intend to do it, and by when they intend to do it. The action plan should be as specific as

Table 6.2.   Profiling example.

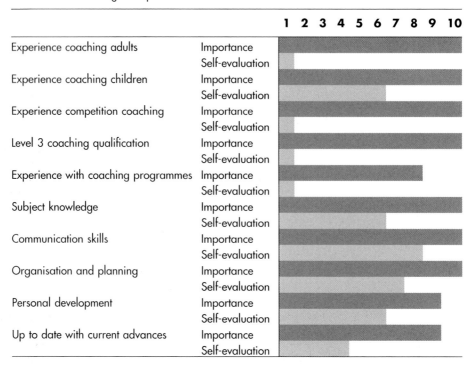

		1 2 3 4 5 6 7 8 9 10
Experience coaching adults	Importance	
	Self-evaluation	
Experience coaching children	Importance	
	Self-evaluation	
Experience competition coaching	Importance	
	Self-evaluation	
Level 3 coaching qualification	Importance	
	Self-evaluation	
Experience with coaching programmes	Importance	
	Self-evaluation	
Subject knowledge	Importance	
	Self-evaluation	
Communication skills	Importance	
	Self-evaluation	
Organisation and planning	Importance	
	Self-evaluation	
Personal development	Importance	
	Self-evaluation	
Up to date with current advances	Importance	
	Self-evaluation	

possible and referred to and updated on a regular basis. Table 6.3 is an example of an action plan.

At this point it is pertinent for the coach to consider the following:

- What am I currently doing and achieving that supports my career goals?
- What barriers are preventing me or may prevent me from reaching my career goals?
- What am I going to do to overcome or pre-empt these barriers?
- What are the next steps I need to undertake to make progress?

Reviewing Progress

One of the keys to successful action planning is to regularly review progress. On a weekly basis the coach should be checking to see if they have achieved or are on the way to achieving the first steps on their action plan and then planning when they are going to take the next steps (they may even decide to have a different action plan each week).

In the longer term it is important to review progress against the main career goal(s). This might be monthly, half yearly, or annually. The purpose is to ensure the main goal is still relevant and exciting. It is quite normal for coaches to change their mind about the direction they want their career to take. It also allows a coach to keep seeing the bigger picture, which is important when day-to-day progress is slow or when they are experiencing setbacks.

Table 6.3.   Example action plan.

Action	How Will You Know When You've Achieved the Action?	First Step	By When	Next Step
Get experience coaching adults	I will be able to include on my C.V. the details of my experience and provide references if required.	Contact local riding clubs to enquire about coaching opportunities.	End of this week	If successful, plan a series of coaching sessions. If not, place an advertisement locally offering freelance tuition.
Get level 3 coaching qualification	I will have completed the course, received a certificate, and be able to include it on my C.V.	Investigate what level 3 coaching qualifications are available, their cost, how long they take to complete, how they are assessed, and what topics they cover.	End of the month	Decide which qualification to pursue.
Get confident and competent in developing and implementing coaching programmes	I will be able to put together coaching programmes for all levels of riders and will be able to provide evidence of the planning and implementation of these programmes.	Look out for any opportunity to develop and implement coaching programmes in my current coaching, for example, Pony Club camp, groups taught in a riding school, individuals who attend regular coaching sessions.	Ongoing	Read up on the theory of planning and implementing coaching programmes.

Figure 6.1 and Table 6.4 illustrate different methods of monitoring progress. Both methods provide a record of the highs and lows over a period of time. The figure is a travelogue, which is a visual representation of progress, and the table is a written progress log.

Another method a coach can employ to monitor their progress in developing their coaching skills is to use a competency-based review. This involves detailing the different competency areas that a coach needs to be able to use and apply and then gathering and recording evidence to chart their progress in developing these areas (Table 6.5). Competency areas could include:

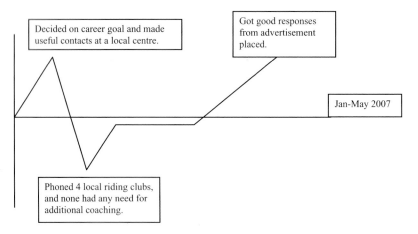

Figure 6.1 Travelogue for reviewing progress.

Table 6.4. Progress log.

Time period: January to May 2007

What Went Well and Why?	What Didn't Go Well and Why?	What Am I Going To Do Differently?
I decided on a career goal and was really excited about it. I spent lots of time auditing my current skills and then researching what was required as a lead coach in an equestrian facility. Made some useful contacts at Elm View Equestrian centre who have offered to help me out if they can. Got good responses to an advertisement I placed in the local tack shop and have now got three new clients, two adults and a teenager.	Phoned all four of the local riding clubs to offer to do some coaching for them, but all felt they had their coaching sessions covered and didn't require anymore at this point in time.	Have a couple of things to work on at any one time so if progress is slow – or nonexistent! – in one area I have something else to focus on.

- The coaching process
- Understanding the individual
- Preparing effective coaching sessions
- Planning and delivering effective coaching sessions

Table 6.5. Example of competency review.

Name:

Competency Area	Requirement	Evidence
Planning and delivering effective coaching session	Be able to prepare activities taking into account riders' needs and motivation.	Log of activities carried out at Pony Club camp and signed by district commissioner.
	Be able to establish a safe working environment	Copy of the risk assessment forms carried out for each activity.
	Be able to set appropriate objectives for coaching sessions	Used Pony Club test guidelines to set appropriate objectives for the level of the group. Copies of the session plans and test guidelines.
	Be able to produce plans for a series of sessions that support riders' development	Produced a scheme of work for the sessions at Pony Club camp that focused on progression of riders towards competition at end. Copy of session plans, activity log, and competition performance.
	Be able to deliver coaching sessions	Delivered two coaching sessions daily for a week at Pony Club camp. Activities included flatwork, show jumping, and cross country. Activity log signed by district commissioner.
	Be able to monitor and evaluate riders' performance and the effectiveness of the sessions	All sessions were evaluated (see session plans) and then a more thorough evaluation was conducted at the end of the week (see reflective journal).
	Be able to effectively conclude the coaching session	At the end of each session all riders were given a summary of the aim of the session and what had been achieved in the session as well as given individual feedback. See activity log signed by district commissioner.
	Be able to monitor and evaluate own coaching practice	Completed evaluation of each session and also evaluated the week's experience highlighting what went well and what I would do differently (see reflective journal).

Note: Ideally, the individual should collect and record a broad range of evidence from different sources and situations.

- Developing a coaching programme
- Managing and developing coaching practice

   In addition to their action plans, progress, or competency reviews a coach should keep a "brag file". This is a place where they can make a note of all the successes they encounter along their journey to coaching excellence. It might include competition results for competitors or teams they have been involved with, a thank you note from someone they coach, a copy of a particularly successful coaching session or coaching programme, or their own written notes about things they have done and are proud of. The benefit of having such a file cannot be understated. Not only will it prove helpful when writing job applications or preparing for interviews, but it also provides a unique record of a coach's progress towards their goals.

SUMMARY

- The primary source of coaching knowledge is coaching experience. However, turning this experience into coaching expertise requires reflection.
- Effective coaches are characterised by a commitment to ongoing learning and reflection.
- There are many different methods of coaching reflection: discussion groups, mentoring, experiential learning, problem-based learning, and keeping a reflective journal.
- All coaches should make time to consider their career goals, conduct a skills audit, and complete a gap analysis or career profile.
- Progress can be reviewed using a travelogue, progress log, or competency review. This should lead to the development of an action plan and brag file.

Self Study

1. Start a reflective journal using the template in Case Study 6.4 (Appendix 18).
2. Consider the questions in the personal action plan section to outline your future career goals.
3. Using the template in Case Study 6.6, complete a coaching skills audit (Appendix 19).
4. Develop a gap analysis to illustrate where you are currently and where you want to be in your coaching career using the template in Appendix 20.
5. Draw up an action plan using the template in Appendix 21.
6. Complete either a travelogue (Appendix 22) or a progress log (Appendix 23) for the last six months.
7. Undertake a competency-based review using the templates in Appendix 24–29.
8. Start a brag file.

Exam Style Questions

1. Describe three different methods of coach reflection.
2. Explain how to use a competency review to chart progress.
3. Discuss the importance of analysing personal coaching practice.

REFERENCES

Cushion, C. (2005). Learning to coach: Linking theory and practice, novice and expert. www.sports-media.org/newpedimensionoctober2005.htm, accessed 27/07/07.

Gilbert, W. and Trudel, P. (1999). Framing the construction of coaching knowledge in experiential learning theory. *Sociology of Sport Online*, 2, www.physed.otago.ac.nz/sosol./home.htm.

Gilbert, W.D. and Trudel, P. (2001). Learning to coach through experience: Reflection in model youth sport coaches. *Journal of Teaching in Physical Education*, 21, 16–34.

Martens, R. (1997). *Successful Coaching*. Champaign, IL: Human Kinetics.

Wallace, S. (2001). *Teaching and Supporting Learning in Further Education*. Exeter: Learning Matters Ltd.

Specialist Coaching

Chapter Objective

To provide an insight into the unique challenges of coaching the disabled rider, the elite rider, and teams.

7.1   THE DISABLED RIDER

Before receiving any coaching all disabled riders should get permission from a doctor to participate, and the coach would be well advised to consult a physiotherapist about the rider's physical abilities. This will ensure they are well-informed and able to choose exercises that will benefit and not harm the rider. It is often an advantage (although not always possible) to have a physiotherapist present during coaching sessions to deal with specific problems as they arise.

There are many reasons for disabled people to ride. Obviously, many are athletes in their own right and compete at the very highest level. There are approximately 80 disabled riders competing in the U.K. today, and 10% of those will be on the elite Paralympic team and a further 12% on the start and potential programmes.

However, riding can also be used as therapy both physically and mentally. Conditions that involve disorders of balance and movement can be helped by using the movement of the horse to initiate a response from the individual. Many disabled riders ride for the remedial effect, improving their balance and coordination both at rest and while moving. Equally, many individuals ride simply for the pleasure of riding. For those people confined to wheelchairs or heavily reliant on others, riding offers psychological benefits and freedom they are otherwise unable to experience.

Classification of Disabled Riders for Competition

Any loss, impairment, or abnormality, whether psychological, physical, or anatomical, classifies the rider as disabled and qualifies them to compete in the Paralympics. Learning difficulties are no longer included as they are hard to measure and subject to different measurements in different countries. The Special Olympics are now run for those who are intellectually disabled, that is, those who have no physical disability, just a learning impairment.

For the Paralympics, riders are profiled individually and not by disease or impairment. They are assessed by a trainer, approved physiotherapist, medical doctor, ophthalmologist, and psychologist. There are five grades that are specific to equine competition:

Ia Most disabled
Ib
II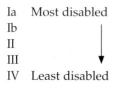
III
IV Least disabled

In equine sports it is the pelvis that is considered the key to classifying disability. The rider is assessed on how good their pelvic tilt is. These assessments are done off the horse, on a bed in a supervised consulting room and with any prosthesis the rider uses.

Those riders who are born disabled will remain in a classification for life unless the disease or disability becomes progressively worse, in which case their classification will change to the next category down (i.e., more severe). This is often the case with multiple sclerosis or cerebral palsy sufferers, who may start in grade IV but progress through the grades as their health deteriorates.

Some athletes have their disability through accident or injury, and often these riders find their mobility returning over time, in which case they move up the classifications (e.g., from II to III).

Multiple sclerosis sufferers are reassessed every six months. However, a rider can request a reassessment or a country or steward can appeal against a classification or request a review.

All riders carry a card with their profile number, disability grade, and any equipment they need to ride with, such as bars or extra reins. Grade I and II riders can have their coach ride their horse for up to 20 minutes before they get on; this is as much a safety consideration as it is a training one. The coach must not ride the horse in the last 15 minutes before it goes into the arena. Grade I and II riders can use their voice, and blind riders use completely boarded arenas – the horses rarely jump out! The dressage tests for each category increase in difficulty from walk only tests up to medium level as illustrated in Table 7.1.

Table 7.1. Requirements of tests for disabled riders.

Grade	
Ia	Walk only
Ib	Walk and trot
II	Walk and trot equivalent to Novice level
III	Walk, trot, and canter equivalent to Elementary level
IV	Walk, trot and canter equivalent to Medium level
Freestyle	Can do more advanced work
	IV can go up to Prix St. Georges
	II can canter and do single flying changes
	Ib can do shoulder in and half pass
	Ia can do walk pirouettes, shoulder in, and half pass

Coaching Guidelines

The disabled rider should be treated in the same way as an able-bodied rider. In fact these riders are often highly driven and motivated, which can lead them to set unrealistic goals. The coach should endeavour to have goals related to personal bests, effort, and improvement. The main goal in coaching riders with a disability is for them to be able to ride a horse to the best of their ability. Clearly, individual's capabilities will vary, but the coach should not be afraid to aim high.

One of the main concerns with novice or inexperienced coaches of riders with disabilities is discussing the disability or impairment. They are often shy, embarrassed, and worried about causing offence. However, the successful coach and rider relationship will be based on open and frank discussion. The riders are the best source of information about what they can and can't do, and the coach should not be reluctant to use this expertise.

Specialist Equipment

All horses or ponies used for disabled riders should wear a breastplate with a leather handle stitched into it. Saddles can also be adapted with a leather strap or metal bar welded onto the tree to prevent the rider from balancing on the horse's mouth. Safety stirrups should be used, and if there is a risk of pressure sores, then a saddle saver can be added.

Some riders who suffer from muscle spasms are better off without stirrups. Velcro or elastic bands can be used to minimise the movement if it is causing problems for the horse or rider. Again, this should only be done after consultation with a physiotherapist. Wheelchair-bound riders will also often use a piece of Velcro glued to the stirrup and the soles of their boots to prevent losing stirrups whilst riding.

Reins can be adapted in many different ways according to the needs of the rider. The most simple adaptation for those riders who find it difficult to tell left from right is to use different colour reins, for example, red for right, blue for left. Most of the ideas for modifications come from the riders themselves who know their problems better than anyone.

Psychology

Socialising is very important for people with disabilities. Discussing problems and ideas and learning to support each other helps them to realise that they are not so different after all.

Physically disabled riders tend to become frustrated when their bodies will not obey them, and success often involves being able to work round or overcoming the problem. Telling a rider who suffers from involuntary muscle spasms to "sit still" or "relax" is simply not helpful. The body may be weak, but this doesn't mean the mind is too. The riders often progress quickly once their understanding of what is required improves, despite their physical limitations. The coach should therefore ensure that they use the same level and depth of technical instructors as they would for all other riders.

Riders with learning difficulties need to be taught differently as they often have no concept of what a circle is – or indeed any other shape – and may find the idea of rising trot hard to grasp. The main goal for these riders is to be stimulated and have fun. Communication is clearly problematical with individuals struggling to express themselves and comprehend what they are being asked to do.

Table 7.2. Physical and learning disabilities.

Condition	Symptoms	Riding Considerations
Down's syndrome	Varying levels of intelligence High incidence of deafness Physical problems Heart abnormalities	Short limbs may lead to problems of balance and control.
Autism	Introverted behaviour Language problems Repetitive movements Intolerance of change Little nonverbal communication	The rhythmic movement of the horse may provide reassurance, and physical contact with the horse may help to develop other relationships.
Blindness	May be partial or complete. May only be able to see short distances May have loss of vision in one or both eyes May have loss of peripheral vision May only be able to see things directly in front (tunnel vision)	Touch and hearing are very important. Speak slowly and continuously when moving so the rider knows where you are. Describe surroundings.
Deafness	Most riders will wear hearing aids and may also lip read and use sign language	Find out how the rider normally communicates. Make eye contact when giving instructions Use a helper to relay instructions.

In particular, the coach should be aware of the following potential limitations of these riders and adapt their coaching accordingly:

- Limited vocabulary and short-term memory
- Poor attention span
- Poor recognition of sequencing
- Possible hearing problems
- Require relaxation time
- Don't understand comparatives, such as longer, bigger, etc.
- Have difficulty discriminating between words, for example, *rein* and *rain*

Table 7.2 provides further information on specific conditions of learning and physical disabilities.

7.2 THE ELITE RIDER

Elite riders are often required to travel to and compete in countries and climates other than the one in which they do most of their training. This raises a number of issues for the coach, not least of which is thermoregulation or the effect of the environment on the performance of both horse and rider.

The Effect of the Environment

Thermoregulation is the ability of the body to control and regulate its core temperature. The core of the body consists of the head, chest, and abdomen. In humans this temperature is 37°C. If it increases or decreases by more than 1°C there will be an effect on the individual's physical and mental performance.

Heat is a by-product of energy metabolism (i.e., converting food to energy), and all muscular contraction produces heat. A small rise in temperature benefits performance by enhancing the power of muscular contraction and ensuring muscles, tendons, and ligaments are more pliable – hence the importance of warming up.

Excessive heat buildup slows energy production, reduces performance, and may be life threatening. Dissipation of heat is therefore an important consideration in both horse and rider, particularly when competing in hot and humid climates.

Heat Transfer

The body can lose or gain heat in four different ways: radiation, conduction, convection, and evaporation. Radiation is the main method of heat loss at rest. When a rider's temperature is greater than the surrounding environment, the heat is lost to cooler objects, such as the floor, walls, and trees.

Conduction occurs when heat is lost through direct transfer from a hotter surface to a cooler one. For example, heat is lost through conduction when a horse is sprayed with cold water or a person immerses themselves in an ice bath.

Convection involves heat exchange via the movement of an air current over the skin. The air picks up the moisture from the skin and carries it away. This occurs when riders stand in a breeze or in front of a fan.

In evaporation heat is used to change a liquid to a vapour. Sweating is the natural process leading to heat loss via evaporation. In hot and humid conditions the riders may sweat, but the sweat does not evaporate into the air because the air is already laden with moisture. This is known as humidity. The sweat runs down the hair on the body in rivulets and drips to the ground. In this case sweating is ineffective at reducing body temperature, and large amounts of fluid and electrolytes are lost.

Factors Affecting Thermoregulation

Factors that affect heat exchange between the horse and rider and the environment include:

- Surface area
- Thickness of coat or clothing
- Environmental temperature
- Relative humidity
- Wind speed

The greater the surface area-to-body weight ratio, the faster heat is lost to the environment. As body size increases, the surface area-to-body weight ratio reduces. This means that small animals lose heat easily but have difficulty staying warm in cold weather. Horses are large with a small surface area, which favours heat retention. Humans, on the other hand, are smaller, with a greater ratio of surface area to body weight, which favours heat loss. The implications are that in hot weather horses are more prone to heat exhaustion than humans. The horse's coat is an insulating layer that reduces heat loss. Clipping is used to facilitate heat loss during exercise but compromises the ability to conserve heat.

In cold weather radiation and conduction are effective at cooling the horse and rider, and they may not even sweat. If the environmental temperature is higher than the body's temperature, then the horse and rider tend to absorb heat by radiation and conduction, making them dependent on convection and evaporation for heat loss.

Low humidity favours evaporation – the drier the air the better it absorbs moisture. High humidity blocks evaporation as the air is already saturated with moisture. This makes sweating relatively ineffective. How fast the air molecules are moving over the skin will also affect heat loss by conduction, convection, and evaporation. The faster the wind speed, the more heat is taken away from the body, which is why large fans are used in countries with both high temperatures and high humidity.

A combination of hot and humid weather is most frequently associated with overheating problems because it reduces the effectiveness of radiation, conduction, and evaporation as methods of losing heat.

Physiological Methods of Heat Loss

The hypothalamus (part of the brain) is the body's internal thermostat. During exercise, the set point of the hypothalamus rises by about 1°C, allowing the muscles to work at their optimum temperature. An increase in blood temperature above this level is a sign that the body is accumulating heat and there is a need to transfer this excess heat to the environment. The body responds as follows.

- **Sweating:** Sweat contains water and electrolytes with a protein (acting as a detergent) to spread the sweat throughout the coat and aid evaporation. When tack rubs against the hair, the detergent is whipped into a white froth.
- **Panting:** Rapid, shallow respirations increase the rate of air flow through the nasal passages. This facilitates heat loss from the blood in the nasal capillaries by conduction, convection, and evaporation.
- **Dilation of cutaneous blood vessels:** The increase in size of the blood vessels nearest the skin increases heat loss by radiation, convection, and evaporation.

One of the benefits of training is that the cooling mechanisms become more efficient. The fitter the horse and rider, the smaller the rise in temperature during exercise.

Monitoring Recovery and Overheating

The horse and rider's recovery from exercise can be monitored and provides a useful indicator of any overheating problems. This monitoring can be done using the following measurements.

- **Heart rate:** Heart rate will decline rapidly during the first few minutes after cessation of exercise, then more slowly. Persistent elevation of the heart rate is indicative of dehydration or exhaustion.
- **Respiratory rate:** This is usually elevated for the first few minutes after exercise, then declines steadily. If the horse or rider needs to lose more heat, they will start to pant.
- **Temperature:** This may continue to rise for the first 5–10 minutes after cessation of exercise but should start to decline within 20–30 minutes.

Dehydration

Dehydration is caused by the loss of water in the body (predominately through sweating) exceeding the fluid intake. Sweating disrupts the electrolyte balance in the body and leads to impaired performance capacity both physically and mentally. The symptoms of dehydration in humans include:

- Headache
- Dizziness/light-headedness
- Nausea and vomiting
- Insomnia
- Irritability
- Impaired mental function
- Tiredness/lethargy
- Muscle fatigue and cramps
- Loss of appetite
- Dark urine

In horses the clinical signs of dehydration include:

- Persistent elevation of the heart and respiratory rate after exercise
- A weak pulse
- Muscular weakness or tremors
- Sunken eyeballs
- Depression
- Dry mouth
- Small amounts of dry faeces
- Reduced urine output

A simple check for dehydration in horses is the skin pinch test. A couple of centimetres of skin over the shoulder is pinched gently between the thumb and finger and then released. In a normally hydrated horse it will ping back rapidly into place. In a seriously dehydrated horse a small residual fold of skin is left longer than expected before returning to its original state.

Avoiding Dehydration

The key to avoiding dehydration is to ensure that both horse and rider are fully hydrated before and during exercise. In humans this is relatively easily achieved by drinking fluids at regular intervals and not waiting for the thirst response before having a drink. Horses can be encouraged to regularly take water by making it more palatable using sugar beet water; soaking hay; feeding sloppy, wet feeds; and allowing free access to water right up to the competition.

After exercise, it is important to replenish the electrolytes lost through sweating. The main electrolytes are sodium (Na), potassium (K), chloride (Cl), calcium (Ca), and phosphorous (P). The most important electrolyte, as far as restoring fluid loss is concerned, is sodium. So by simply adding small amounts of salt to a rider's water bottle or a horse's feed (or free access to a salt lick if the horse will use one) goes a long way to combating dehydration.

Acclimatisation

Both horses and riders will cope much better with hot or humid conditions after 10–14 days of daily exercise in such conditions. In the first 2–4 days there may be symptoms of tiredness and depression, but by days 5 and 6 there should begin to be an improvement. Acclimatisation will not compensate fully for the effects of heat and humidity, but it should increase exercise tolerance and reduce the risk of heat-related disorders.

Prior to travelling to competitions in hot and humid conditions, many riders attempt to start their acclimatisation period in this country by exercising in several layers of clothes and putting exercise rugs on their horses.

Cooling Methods

Cold water cooling is a useful method of rapidly cooling down hot horses, speeding recovery, and reducing the chances of heat stress. This technique involves using convection and evaporation to facilitate heat loss.

Ideally, a shady spot is needed, along with several buckets of water and large blocks of ice. Immediately after exercise, the cold water is applied liberally to all parts of the body, including the quarters. Excess water is not scraped off and the cold water should keep being applied and alternated with 20–30 seconds of walking in a circle. Walking promotes blood flow to the skin and therefore encourages cooling by convection. The movement of air aids cooling through evaporation.

The horse's temperature should be checked at regular intervals. It should fall by around 1°C in 10 minutes. Allow the horse to drink small amounts of water (half a bucket) during the competition and immediately after exercise. This will help cool the horse and reduce dehydration. Stop cooling if:

- The rectal temperature falls below 38–39°C
- The skin over the quarters feels cold to the touch after a walking period
- The respiratory rate is less than 30 breaths per minute

The rider can also take measures to avoid heat stress. Removing the hat, sitting in the shade, and washing the face with cold water are all effective ways of reducing body temperature. They should also be encouraged to drink an isotonic drink. Ideally, the rider competing in hot climates should wear light-coloured (preferably white), loose fitting, cotton clothing.

Things to avoid include:

- Putting ice against the skin, as this reduces cooling by stopping blood flow to the area under the pack
- Putting wet towels on the horse, as they soon warm up and act as insulation preventing heat loss
- Excessive application of grease prior to cross country limits sweating, as it too acts as insulation
- Letting horses stand still for prolonged periods
- Restricting a horse's access to water before and during competition
- Giving the horse ice cold water to drink

Exercising in a Cold Climate

Competitions are seldom held in extremely cold conditions, although many horses will continue to be exercised when the weather is cold. Horses undergoing strenuous exercise at –25°C have been shown to have no significant changes in heart rate, lactate production (lactic acid), gait, or lung tissue morphology (composition). The only difference is a reduction in the respiratory rate at all stages of exercise and recovery as the cold temperature facilitates heat loss. The main consideration for exercising horses in cold weather is the increased amount of time required in the warm-up and the condition of the ground.

In humans the effect of a cold environment on exercise performance depends largely on the severity of the temperature and the type of exercise being performed. In fact, exposure to a moderately cold environment can actually improve performance as the cardiovascular system no longer has to divert blood to the periphery for heat loss. This results in less stress being placed on the heart. However, exposure to extreme cold may cause the body's core temperature to drop, and hence an athlete's aerobic capacity will be reduced, which will impair their performance.

Nutritional Considerations

At the elite level the horse and rider are required to perform at their optimum levels. This requires the ability to effectively and efficiently produce energy for movement. In order to ensure the right amount and type of energy is available the coach needs to pay close attention to the nutritional intakes of both horse and rider.

The Rider

Our diets consist of macronutrients (required in large quantities) and micronutrients (required in small quantities). The main energy-providing macronutrients are:

- Carbohydrates
- Fat
- Protein

Fibre, water, vitamins, and minerals are also essential in the diet but provide no energy.

In terms of energy requirement, a sedentary person should have a diet divided into approximately 50% carbohydrates, 20% protein, and 30% fat. However, in order for a sports person to meet their energy requirements the division should be nearer 65% carbohydrates, 15% protein, and 20% fat. Before a competition this is likely to increase to 70% from carbohydrate, 15% from protein, and 15% from fat (Figure 7.1).

Carbohydrates are important because they fuel the brain and the central nervous system as well as the muscles. Simple carbohydrates are broken down quickly, so they help with short-term energy. Complex carbohydrates take longer to break down so are good for sustained energy throughout the day. Table 7.3 provides examples of both simple and complex carbohydrate-containing foods.

Table 7.3. Foods containing carbohydrates.

Simple Carbohydrates (sugary)	Complex Carbohydrates (starchy)
Jam and marmalade	Bread
Syrup and treacle	Pasta and noodles
Boiled sweets	Potatoes
Biscuits	Pulses and legumes – peas, lentils, beans
Jellies	Dried fruit
Pancakes	Baked beans
Lucozade	Fresh fruit – apples, pears, oranges, grapes, bananas
Fruit yoghurt	Cereal – Weetabix, shredded wheat
Jaffa Cakes	Porridge
Chocolate	Sugar-free muesli
Fig rolls	Popcorn
Fruit crumble	Rice

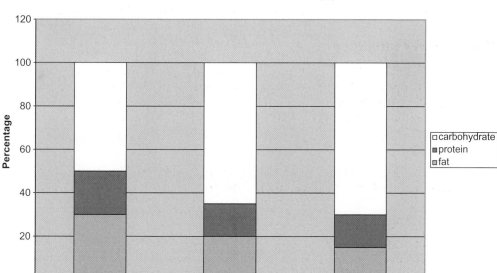

Figure 7.1   Dietary split of macronutrients.

Fat also plays an important role in the human body by:

- Protecting internal organs
- Providing insulation
- Storing energy
- Metabolising fat-soluble vitamins
- Helping to maintain a healthy nervous system

However, not all fats are equal. Saturated fats (those that are solid at room temperature) are generally from animals and can cause deposits in the arteries. Unsaturated fats (liquid at room temperature) are generally derived from plants and can be mono- or polyunsaturated. The fat part of our diet should be high in mono- and polyunsaturated fats and low in saturated fats.

Protein is essential for building and repairing muscles and other tissues as well as synthesising hormones and should contribute between 12 and 15% of the total daily calorie intake. Examples of high-protein foods include:

- Eggs
- Meat and poultry
- Fish
- Legumes
- Dairy products
- Tofu
- Nuts
- Bread and rice

Table 7.4. Types of vitamins.

Water Soluble	Fat Soluble
Vitamin B complex	Vitamin A, D, E, and K
Vitamin C	

Table 7.5. Minerals and trace elements.

Minerals	Trace Elements
Calcium	Iron
Potassium	Zinc
Sodium	Copper
	Selenium

Vitamins are essential to the normal functioning of the body even though they are not a source of energy. They help to regulate the chemical reactions in the body, and an absence or deficiency of vitamins can lead to disease. There are two types of vitamins, water-soluble and fat-soluble (Table 7.4). Minerals and trace elements also perform vital functions within the body but they are only required in small amounts (Table 7.5).

Fibre is found in the outer walls of plants and seeds. It provides the non-energy bulk that is essential to the proper functioning of the gut. Water is another essential element in the diet. It has a role in:

- Cellular function
- Stabilising body temperature
- Carrying nutrients and waste

Energy Balance

To maintain body weight the rider needs to be in energy balance. This means that their energy intake (food and drink) is equal to their energy expenditure (activity and exercise). For men this is usually around 2,500 kcal/day and for women 2,000 kcal/day.

In some sports (such as racing) a low body weight is an advantage or even essential, and unhealthy weight loss techniques are undertaken that can be detrimental to both the health of the rider and their performance. These include:

- Food restriction, including fasting, vomiting, laxatives, appetite suppressants, diet pills
- Drastic dehydration, including fluid restriction and use of diuretics, sauna, rubber suit, exercising in heat
- Enemas
- Over-exercising
- Nose bleeding and blood letting

The best way to ensure that weight loss is done in a controlled, sustainable, and healthy manner is to stick to the following guidelines:

- Decrease energy intake by no more than 500 kcal/day.
- Energy intake should not go below 1,500 kcal/day.
- Lose no more than 0.5kg/week.
- Increase the amount of energy from carbohydrate and reduce the amount of energy from fat.
- Include aerobic exercise in the training programme to promote fat loss and increase energy expenditure.

The Horse

The intestinal tract of the horse is highly developed to extract nutrients from the digestion of plant matter. This roughage (hay or grass) acts as the foundation upon which to build a feeding programme. The high fibre content of roughage is essential to normal intestinal function and therefore the health of the horse.

Metabolism of roughage in the large intestine and the fermentation and breakdown of fibre generate large amounts of VFA (volatile fatty acids). These, as well as sugars (glucose), can be used immediately for energy or are stored as fat.

The following are guidelines for best meeting the horse's nutritional requirements:

- The horse can only consume 2.5% of its body weight per day in feed (concentrate and roughage).
- At least 50% of the daily ration (by weight) should consist of roughage.
- The higher the proportion of roughage, the "safer" (less risk of disease such as laminitis, colic, and limb deformities in youngsters) the diet for the horse.
- Measure all feed by weight not volume; the weights of different bales of hay and different concentrates varies.
- Feed at regular intervals and ideally at the same time every day.
- Allow free access to hay.

As with the rider, the horse's primary source of energy is carbohydrate, which is found in the fibre components of hay and grass as well as in concentrate feeds.

Fat is an excellent source of energy for those horses working aerobically (speeds less than 12mph and heart rates less than 150 beats per minute). However, only 12–15% of a ration should be fed in the form of fat. Vegetable oil is a useful fat supplement for endurance horses and those working for long periods of time at slow speeds.

Protein is commonly overfed to horses. Protein will only be used as an energy source if there is a lack of carbohydrates or fats. Mature horses require only moderate amounts of protein (8–10% of the ration). Growing horses and pregnant or lactating mares may need up to 16% of the ration as protein.

Weight loss strategies for the horse are similar to those for the rider. Weight loss should be gradual and should not include restricting access to roughage. Instead, the horse should have high-energy foods substituted for less energy-rich foodstuffs by eliminating concentrates and oil and replacing them with hay and moving from rich pastures. A suitable aerobic fitness programme will also help to increase the energy expenditure.

7.3 TEAM SPORTS

Some coaches will be heavily involved in coaching teams throughout their career whilst others may only periodically be involved with their local Pony Club or Riding Club teams. In team sports such as horseball and polo group, cohesion is an important consideration. Cohesion is concerned with the extent to which a team is willing to stick together and work together. There are two areas that tend to influence members to remain within a team: task cohesion and social cohesion.

Task cohesion is the degree to which the team members are committed to achieving common goals, such as winning tournaments or beating the opposition. Social cohesion is the degree to which the team members like each other, get on well, and trust and support each other.

Building Group Cohesion

Davis et al (2005) suggest that in order to perform at its potential, a team needs to ensure that it makes the best use of the ability of its individual members (task cohesion) as well as maximising team cooperation (social cohesion). This can be done by:

- Making the team distinct (team name, kit, slogans, and songs)
- Having clear group and individual goals that are shared and accepted
- Having clear formal roles (e.g., team captain) and recognition of informal roles (e.g., team motivator) performed by individuals in the team
- Encouraging shared decision making where appropriate
- Developing mutual respect
- Ensuring training is fun and interactive as well as individually challenging

In addition, Yukelson (1997) suggested that coaches have a key role in the development of an effective team culture and that they could influence it through:

- Getting to know their athletes as unique individuals
- Developing pride in group membership and a sense of team identity
- Developing team goals and team commitment (e.g., most consistent team/most hard-working team in the league, etc.)
- Evaluating goals periodically, charting progress, and seeking and providing feedback
- Clarifying roles, helping all individuals to feel valued and building mutual understanding
- Having periodic team meetings to discuss progress openly and honestly
- Keeping informed of attitudes and feelings within the team through meetings with individuals, team representatives or the captain, or small groups of team members

Self Study

1. Visit a local Riding for the Disabled (RDA) centre, dressage competition for disabled riders, or a coaching session for disabled riders. Make notes on:
    *   Any specialist equipment and tack you can see being used and what its purpose is.
    *   Different approaches to training and riding and comment on why this approach might have been adopted and its benefits.
    *   Exercises used to improve balance, coordination, and to help the rider to ride to the best of their ability.
    *   The language of the trainer: Do they use different expressions to help explain movements and exercises?

    Ideally, you should aim to observe disabled riders being trained for competition as well as riding being used as therapy and life enhancement for disabled people.

2. Ask one of the riders you coach to keep a log of their food intake for a week.
    *   Assess the quantities of carbohydrate, fat, and protein that make up the diet.
    *   Compare and contrast the log with the suggested percentages in Figure 7.1.
    *   Plan a daily menu for the next week using the information provided in this chapter.

3. Outline an action plan for improving team cohesion.
    *   Include specific activities to be undertaken by the team as a whole and activities that focus on the individual members of the team, as well as particular actions that the coach should undertake.

REFERENCES

Davis, B., Roscoe, J., Roscoe, D. and Bull, B. (2005). *Physical Education and the Study of Sport*. Edinburgh: Elsevier Ltd.

Yukelson, D. (1997). Principles of effective team building intervention in sport: A direct services approach at Penn State University. *Journal of Applied Sport Psychology, 9*, 73–96.

Appendix 1
Goal-Setting Template

Rider: Standard:		
Long-Term Aim		
Long-Term Goal		
Intermediate Goal		
Intermediate Goal		
Intermediate Goal		
Intermediate Goal		
	Goal	**Time Frame**
Intermediate Goal		
Short-term goal		
Short-term goal		
Short-term goal		
Short-term goal		
Short-term goal		
Short-term goal		
Goal Evaluation		
Goal		
Completed by		
Outcome		
Evaluation		

Appendix 2
Performance Profiling Template

Characteristic / Skill		1	2	3	4	5	6	7	8	9	10
	Importance										
	Self-evaluation										
	Importance										
	Self-evaluation										
	Importance										
	Self-evaluation										
	Importance										
	Self-evaluation										
	Importance										
	Self-evaluation										
	Importance										
	Self-evaluation										
	Importance										
	Self-evaluation										
	Importance										
	Self-evaluation										
	Importance										
	Self-evaluation										
	Importance										
	Self-evaluation										

Characteristic / Skill		1	2	3	4	5	6	7	8	9	10
	Role Model										
	Self-evaluation										
	Role Model										
	Self-evaluation										
	Role Model										
	Self-evaluation										
	Role Model										
	Self-evaluation										
	Role Model										
	Self-evaluation										
	Role Model										
	Self-evaluation										
	Role Model										
	Self-evaluation										
	Role Model										
	Self-evaluation										
	Role Model										
	Self-evaluation										
	Role Model										
	Self-evaluation										

Appendix 3
Scorecard for Fitness Tests

Test	Score 1 Date:	Score 2 Date:	Score 3 Date:
Resting heart rate			
Sit-ups			
Sit and reach test			
Stork stand			
Hand, ball, wall test			

Appendix 4
Fitness Demands Profile

Discipline	
Duration of event	
Demands: CV fitness	
Muscular strength	
Muscular endurance	
Flexibility	
Body composition	
Balance	
Co-ordination	
Reaction time	
Speed and agility	

Appendix 5
Circuit Training Template

Exercise	Number of Repetitions

Appendix 6
Training Programme Template

Horse: Level:			
Frequency	Intensity	Time	Type
Week no:			
Week no:			
Week no:			
Week no:			
Weeks no:			
Rider: **Level:**			
Frequency	Intensity	Time	Type
Week no:			
Week no:			

Appendix 7
Risk Assessment Template

Date: **Session type:** **Venue:** **No of riders:** **Level:**	
Rider	Check experience – during introduction
	Check experience with current horse – introduction
	Check competence – observe warm-up
Horse	Check experience – during introduction
	Assess temperament – observe warm-up
	Assess suitability for rider – observe warm-up
Activity	Check equipment – on arrival
	Assess suitability of session plan – after warm-up
Environment	Check ground conditions/surface – on arrival
	Assess weather conditions/lighting – on arrival
	Assess suitability for session – on arrival
Equipment	Check poles, stands, cups – on arrival
	Check cross country fences – on arrival
	Check boards/markers – on arrival
	Check tack – during introduction
	Check appropriate clothing/equipment – introduction
Coaching Method	Assess suitability for all horses and riders – after warm-up
Supervision	Appropriate ratio rider/coach – on arrival
	Appropriate medical/vet cover – on arrival
	Appropriate first aid cover – on arrival
	Appropriate first aid equipment – on arrival
Review Notes	

Risk Identified	Risk Evaluation	Action

Appendix 8
Accident Report Form

Date:	Rider name:
Time:	Horse name:
Place:	Activity:

Nature of injury:

What happened:

Action taken:

Appendix 9
Session Plan

Rider: Horse:	
Date	
Objective	
Learning Assessment	
Prerequisites	
Facilities	
Equipment/resources	

Activity
    Intro
    (minutes)
    Warm-up
    (minutes)	

Review previous (minutes)	
Main activity (minutes)	
Practice (minutes)	
Review (minutes)	
Evaluation/comments	

Appendix 10
Scheme of Work

Scheme of work: **Syllabus:**
Date: **Group:**

Day	Time	Practical/Theory	Topic	Resources	Private Study/Practice

Appendix 11
Competition Plan

Competition	
Date	
Venue	
Horse/Rider	
Objective(s)	
Evaluation	

Appendix 12
Team Selection Plan

Team	
Main Competition	
Date	
Venue	
Objective(s)	
Short-listed Riders	
Team Selection Criteria	
Team Selection Deadline	
Team Training Details (dates and venues)	

Appendix 13
Team Plan

Team	
Competition	
Date	
Venue	
Objective(s)	
Team Riders + Reserve	

Name of Rider and Horse	Riding Order	Individual Objective(s)

Team Tactics/Strategy

Appendix 14
Individual Learning Plan

Name:	Age:
Height:	Weight:
Any limiting factors (medical issues/disabilities)	
Riding Experience	
Competition Experience	
Fitness Levels	
Aspirations	
Current Ability	
Riding position	
Jumping position	
Effectiveness on flat/over fences	
Care of the horse	
Training of the horse	
Psychological skills	
Attitude	
Strengths	
Areas for improvement	

Appendix 15
Show Jumping Analysis Template

S/US

Fence 1

S/US

Fence 2

S/US

Fence 3

S/US

Fence 4

S/US

Fence 5

S/US

Fence 6

S/US

Fence 7

S/US

Fence 8

S/US

Fence 9

S/US

Fence 10

S/US

Fence 11

S/US

Fence 12

Appendix 16
Dressage Warm-Up Analysis

Rider & Horse:
Date:
Level of test:
Score:

Venue:
Test number:
Placing:

Warm-up Start Time		Warm-up Finish Time		Total Warm-up Time	

Walk

Start Time	Finish Time	Movements Performed	Number of Minutes

Total time

Trot

Start Time	Finish Time	Movements Performed	Number of Minutes

Total time

Canter

Start Time	Finish Time	Movements Performed	Number of Minutes

Total time

Appendix 17
Analysis of a Fence on a Cross Country Course

Competiton: **Date:**
Class: **No of**
Fence: **Competitors:**

Competitor	Direct Route	Alternative Route	Outcome	Time Taken
1				
2				
3				
4				
5				
6				
7				
8				
9				
10				
11				
12				
13				

14				
15				
16				
17				
18				
19				
20				

Appendix 18
Reflective Journal Template

Session:	
Date:	
What went well and why?	
What didn't go well and why?	
What would I do differently?	

What have I learnt about:
  1. myself
  2. my subject knowledge
  3. my coaching skills
  4. the riders/horses	

How can I apply what I have learnt?	
What do I need to learn more about?	
What am I going to do next?	1. 2. 3.

Appendix 19
Skills Audit Template

Coaching Skills	Communication	
	Planning	
	Feedback	
	Reflection	
Knowledge	Developing horses	
	Developing riders	
	Sports psychology	
	Horse behaviour	
Experience	Coaching children	
	Discipline-Specific	

Appendix 20
Career Profiling Template

		1	2	3	4	5	6	7	8	9	10
	Importance										
	Self-evaluation										
	Importance										
	Self-evaluation										
	Importance										
	Self-evaluation										
	Importance										
	Self-evaluation										
	Importance										
	Self-evaluation										
	Importance										
	Self-evaluation										
	Importance										
	Self-evaluation										
	Importance										
	Self-evaluation										
	Importance										
	Self-evaluation										
	Importance										
	Self evaluation										
	Importance										
	Self-evaluation										
	Importance										
	Self-evaluation										
	Importance										
	Self-evaluation										

Appendix 21
Action Plan Template

Action	How Will You Know When You've Achieved the Action?	First Step	By When	Next Step

Appendix 22
Travelogue Template

Timescale:

Appendix 23
Progress Log Template

Time period:

What went well and why?	What didn't go well and why?	What am I going to do differently?

Appendix 24
Planning and Delivering Effective Coaching Sessions Competency Review

Name:

Competency Area	Requirement	Evidence
Planning and delivering effective coaching session	Be able to set appropriate objectives for coaching sessions	
	Be able to produce plans for a series of sessions that support riders' development	
	Be able to deliver coaching sessions	
	Be able to monitor and evaluate riders' performance and the effectiveness of the sessions	
	Be able to effectively conclude the coaching session	
	Be able to monitor and evaluate own coaching practice	

Appendix 25
Understanding the Coaching Process Competency Review

Name:

Competency Area	Requirement	Evidence
Understanding the coaching process	Be able to prepare individuals for the coaching process	
	Be able to use appropriate coaching styles, communication, and feedback techniques in coaching sessions	
	Be able to communicate effectively the purpose, goals, and detail of the sessions	
	Be able to check individuals' levels of experience, ability, and motivation to participate	
	Be able to provide effective explanations and demonstrations of techniques	
	Be able to provide and encourage constructive feedback	
	Be able to communicate effectively information about future sessions	
	Be able to use a range of coaching styles and techniques to encourage personal responsibility and decision making in individuals	

Appendix 26
Understanding the Individual Competency Review

Name:

Competency Area	Requirement	Evidence
Understanding the individual	Be able to contribute to the evaluation of participants	
	Be able to explain the needs of a range of individuals	
	Be able to set goals for coaching sessions that meet the needs and aspirations of individuals	
	Be able to prioritise individuals' performance needs using information gathered from a variety of sources	
	Be able to use a range of methods to motivate and encourage individuals	
	Be able to adapt their style to the changing needs of the individual	

Preparing Effective Coaching Sessions Competency Review

Name:

Competency Area	Requirement	Evidence
Preparing effective coaching sessions	Be able to prepare activities, taking into account riders' needs and motivation	
	Be able to establish a safe working environment	
	Be able to prepare the use of appropriate resources to support coaching sessions	
	Be able to prepare appropriate timings, sequences, volume, and intensity of coaching sessions	
	Be able to explain and implement governing body and good practice guidelines	

Appendix 28
Developing a Coaching Programme Competency Review

Name:

Competency Area	Requirement	Evidence
Developing a coaching programme	Be able to review individuals' current and potential needs	
	Be able to identify key factors that influence performance	
	Be able to produce plans for a coaching programme that supports individuals' development	
	Be able to monitor and evaluate a coaching programme	
	Be able to monitor and evaluate individuals' performance	
	Be able to apply training principles and methods to develop individuals' performance	
	Be able to use appropriate methods to analyse individuals' performance	
	Be able to manage the human and physical resources required to support the coaching programme	

Appendix 29
Managing and Developing Coaching Practice Competency Review

Name:

Competency Area	Requirement	Evidence
Managing and developing coaching practice	Continuously develop personal practice	
	Be able to effectively reflect on progress and achievement	
	Be able to identify strengths and areas for improvement	
	Be able to analyse current coaching practice using information from a variety of sources	
	Be able to draw up and implement a personal action	
	Be able to assist others in developing their own coaching practice	
	Be able to recognise and implement advances in coaching and equine knowledge	

Index